Foundation in Pharmacy Practice

Foundation in Pharmacy Practice

Ben J Whalley BPharm (Hons), MRPharmS, PhD

Lecturer in Clinical Pharmacy, Reading School of Pharmacy, University of Reading, UK

Kate E Fletcher MRPharmS, Dip Clin Pharm, PhD

Teacher Practitioner, Reading School of Pharmacy, University of Reading, UK
Lead Pharmacist for Specialist Surgery, Royal Berkshire NHS Foundation Trust, Reading, UK

Sam E Weston MRPharmS, MBA

Teacher Practitioner, Reading School of Pharmacy, University of Reading, UK

Rachel L Howard MRPharmS, Dip Clin Pharm, PhD

Lecturer in Pharmacy Practice, Reading School of Pharmacy, University of Reading, UK

Clare F Rawlinson MPharm, MRPharmS, PhD

Lecturer in Pharmacy Practice, Reading School of Pharmacy, University of Reading, UK

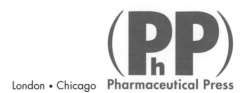

London • Chicago   **Pharmaceutical Press**

Published by the Pharmaceutical Press
An imprint of RPS Publishing

1 Lambeth High Street, London SE1 7JN, UK
100 South Atkinson Road, Suite 200, Greyslake, IL 60030-7820, USA

© Pharmaceutical Press 2008

(**PP**) is a trade mark of RPS Publishing

RPS Publishing is the publishing organisation of the Royal
Pharmaceutical Society of Great Britain

First published 2008

Typeset by J&L Composition Ltd, Filey, North Yorkshire
Printed in Great Britain by Cambridge University Press, Cambridge

ISBN 978 0 85369 747 3

A catalogue record for this book is available from the British Library.

The authors dedicate this book to Dr R T Gladwell, Director of Teaching and Learning, Reading School of Pharmacy (2005–2007)

Contents

Foreword

Many Schools of Pharmacy now introduce Pharmacy Practice at the start of the course to show students how Practice draws on clinical and scientific knowledge and to instil a professional attitude from the very beginning. More practically, students often take vacation and Saturday jobs in a pharmacy to supplement their income as well as to gain experience and they need the basics behind them to do so. Introducing Practice at such an early stage means it is necessary to start at a fundamental level. Until now there has not been a suitable textbook to help the students or their teachers.

The authors, all members of the Pharmacy Practice team at Reading, have experience of the Practice of pharmacy in all its guises: from managing – and owning – a community pharmacy and a locum agency, ethics committee membership, PCT experience, and specialist clinical pharmacy, right through to pre-registration tutelage in both the hospital and community sectors. They have already brought their experience to bear in devising a fresh approach to a new course, in a new School of Pharmacy. The introductory module proved so popular with students that this textbook, including all the new material the team had written, was suggested.

The scope of the book covers the structure of the NHS and RPSGB; the varied and changing roles of the pharmacist in different sectors (including industry); an introduction to medicines management, law, ethics, confidentiality and duty of care; essential communication skills; major routes of drug administration; a very useful section on dispensing: practicalities, labelling, legal issues relating to different types of prescriptions and a beginners guide (with handy tips) to extemporaneous dispensing and routes of administration; and a glossary of commonly used Pharmacy Practice terms.

Foundation in Pharmacy Practice is not only a textbook but it is also a teaching and learning resource, providing checklists, hints and tips. Teachers of Pharmacy Practice will find it useful for developing undergraduate courses, and pre-registration pharmacists will find it a valuable resource and revision guide, as will pharmacists returning to practice after a break, or those moving sector, from hospital to community pharmacy for example. Most importantly, it will help the new undergraduate pharmacy student to discover and find their way around the profession they have chosen.

Elizabeth M Williamson, MRPharmS
Professor of Pharmacy and Director of Practice
April 2008

About the authors

Ben J Whalley

Dr Whalley is a lecturer at the Reading School of Pharmacy. In May 2006 he received an award for outstanding contributions to teaching and learning support from the University of Reading for his part in formulating and delivering the new Pharmacy Practice course, and in particular the development of novel teaching methods, including lecture podcasting and extensive use of the virtual learning environment. He is a qualified and registered pharmacist (1992), and obtained his PhD (Neuroscience) from the School of Pharmacy, University of London in 2003. He continues to practise in the community sector as a registered pharmacist, has worked as a practice-based pharmacist for Bromley Primary Care Trust and has appeared as a scientific adviser in a number of television programmes. He also acts as Receiving Editor for the *European Journal of Neuroscience* and is an Expert Pharmacist Member of the Thames Valley Multi-Centre NHS Research Ethics Committee and an Associate of the Institute of Health Sciences.

Kate E Fletcher

Since qualifying as a pharmacist in 1995, Kate Fletcher has worked in hospital pharmacy, specialising in general surgery, neurosurgery, neuro-intensive care and geratology. She has worked at the Royal Berkshire NHS Foundation Trust in Reading for 4 years, and is currently Lead Pharmacist for Specialist Surgery. She has been involved with teaching nurses, doctors and pharmacists for the past 7 years and has been a pre-registration pharmacist tutor for the past 3 years, tutoring individual trainees and taking part in delivery of the Thames Valley Regional Programme for Pre-Registration Pharmacists. She joined the Department of Pharmacy Practice at the Reading School of Pharmacy in November 2005, where she is involved in developing MPharm course content, lectures on a variety of clinical and non-clinical subjects and supervises practical sessions.

Sam E Weston

Sam Weston currently convenes Year 2 of the Pharmacy Practice course of the School of Pharmacy at the University of Reading, and has played a part in creating and delivering the new undergraduate MPharm course since January 2006. She is a qualified and registered pharmacist (1998), and is currently reading for her PhD at Reading School of Pharmacy, investigating the potential use of cannabis in the treatment of epilepsy. She has an MBA (Open University) and also runs a locum pharmacy agency, whilst continuing to work as a locum pharmacist in the community, hospital and prison sectors.

Rachel L Howard

Rachel Howard has worked as a clinical pharmacist for 10 years in both hospital and general practice, with particular experience in cardiology, care of the elderly and medical admissions.

Since 2000 she has conducted research into the underlying causes of medication-related admissions to hospital and how these events can be avoided. This formed the basis for her PhD, awarded by the University of Nottingham in 2006. Dr Howard has contributed chapters to two books on patient safety, focusing on medicines management in primary care and the exploration of medication-related morbidity. She has worked with leading academics in the field of patient safety, helping to develop a draft design specification for electronic prescribing for NHS prescribing systems and to test an IT-based pharmacist-led intervention to reduce potentially hazardous prescribing in primary care. In 2006 she took up the position of Lecturer in Pharmacy Practice at the University of Reading School of Pharmacy.

Clare F Rawlinson

Dr Rawlinson is a qualified and registered pharmacist (2002) who obtained her PhD in Drug Delivery at the Institute of Pharmaceutical Innovation, University of Bradford (2006). Her experience spans industrial, hospital and community sectors of pharmacy and she previously held a Developmental Lectureship in Pharmaceutics at the University of Bradford. She has recently developed the Law and Ethics module of the Pharmacy Practice course at Reading School of Pharmacy, where her other roles include pre-registration placement tutor and Industrial Pharmacists Group representative. She is a committee member of the Analytical Science Network, which provides support for early career analytical scientists working in all sectors of industry, and which is affiliated with the Analytical Division of the Royal Society of Chemistry. Dr Rawlinson is also a reviewer for the *International Journal of Pharmaceutics*.

Acknowledgements

The writing of any textbook is not conceived or conducted by the authors in glorious isolation. We would therefore like to thank all of the people who have freely given advice, support and time to this endeavour. Moreover, we would also like to thank some particular individuals, without whose efforts this process would have been much harder, if not impossible: Professor E Williamson for her support and advice throughout the writing of this book, and Kevin Flint, David Allen and Daniel Grant for their help with photographs, figures and information sources. Also, many thanks to staff and patients at the Royal Berkshire NHS Foundation Trust for agreeing to have their photographs taken, in particular Mr W G V Woodley, Claire-Louise Cartwright, Jennifer Cockerell, Dr Chloe Dallimore, Tania Jones, Adella Mutero, Sawsan Turkie, Amanda Wheeler and Jonathan Yazbek. We would also like to thank Dr Claudia Vincenzi and Dr Riddhi Shukla for their contributions about careers in industrial pharmacy.

Finally, we should not forget that large parts of the Pharmacy Practice courses that we teach are influenced significantly by the students we are privileged to teach. Their enthusiasm for, commitment to and engagement with our courses provide constant inspiration and motivation in our work, which we hope is reflected in this book.

1

What is Pharmacy Practice?

Ben J Whalley

Introduction

The principal aim of this book is to provide an essential reference on Pharmacy Practice for Pharmacy Masters (MPharm) students, particularly those just embarking on their study of Pharmacy at undergraduate level. As such, it provides an overview of the major topics in Pharmacy Practice encountered by such students, in a practical, clear and succinct manner.

As a text aimed at new Pharmacy students, it is not intended as an exhaustive reference text for each topic covered; rather, it should be considered as a starting point for further study, facilitated by regular signposting and referencing to the many excellent advanced texts available. Students are strongly encouraged to pursue such directions as required, and as their overall level of understanding and ability develops.

The rapidly changing nature of the profession and the unfamiliar terminology and acronyms that are widely used often present barriers to students beginning their study of Pharmacy Practice. This book provides a glossary of common terms used in the discipline, which can be used either as the book is read as a whole, or as a companion text during the study of other texts on Pharmacy Practice.

This book also provides a practical guide to extemporaneous dispensing, including hints and tips for successful dispensing. This guide is to be used in conjunction with formal pharmaceutical texts such as:

- *British Pharmacopoeia* (BP)
- *British National Formulary* (*BNF*; published every 6 months)
- *Martindale: The Complete Drug Reference*
- *Pharmaceutical Codex*
- *Medicines, Ethics and Practice Guide for Pharmacists and Pharmacy Technicians* (MEP; published annually).

Pharmacy Practice: definitions

As a first step in undertaking the study of Pharmacy Practice, it is vital to understand what the term means. What is Pharmacy Practice? Which specific subject areas does it encompass? How does it relate and link to other relevant disciplines that comprise the undergraduate Pharmacy degree? Considering and answering these important questions will provide an overview of the subject, a prerequisite for its successful study and practice.

In simple terms, Pharmacy Practice is the discipline within Pharmacy that involves developing the professional roles of the pharmacist. Consequently, and within the scope of the MPharm degree, it can also be described as *application* of the knowledge and skills acquired as part of the other related disciplines within the MPharm programme to actual patient care.

By giving careful consideration to the definition above, it should be clear that a solid grasp of Pharmacy Practice is vital, since it facilitates and enables pharmacists to fully exploit their substantial knowledge and expertise in areas such as pharmacology, pharmaceutics, chemistry and therapeutics within a clinical context.

More than a definition

Whilst the definition used above provides us with the scope of the discipline, it is also important to consider the individual components that comprise the whole. The following areas can be considered as critical parts of the discipline.

Healthcare systems

To operate effectively and deliver the best care to patients, a pharmacist needs to understand the way in which healthcare provision to the general population is organised in the UK. A pharmacist should be able to comprehensively answer questions such as:

- Which public and private organisations deliver healthcare to the population?
- Which professionals work in which areas to provide such health care?
- What role does the UK Government play in such provision?
- How do individual patients enter such systems for treatment?

As one of the largest employers in Europe, the UK's National Health Service (NHS) has enormous scope and size, making the answers to the above questions important. An overview of past and current NHS structure and healthcare provision is provided in Chapter 2.

Public health (*Chapter 2*)

As health professionals, pharmacists are concerned not just with the treatment of existing disease states, but also with their prevention and the promotion of healthier lifestyles. Consequently, the area of public health concerns the prevention rather than the treatment of disease, often via the surveillance of specific disease states and the promotion of healthy behaviours shown to reduce the incidence and/or severity of such states. This has given rise to a definition of public health as the science and art of promoting health, preventing disease and prolonging healthy life through the organised efforts of society.

The role of the pharmacist (*see Chapters 3–5*)

Many students entering the study of Pharmacy are already aware of the traditional role of the pharmacist as a dispenser of medicines prescribed by doctors and other health professionals; however, it is critical to appreciate that the pharmacist's role has developed rapidly in recent years to include many other roles beyond the dispensing of drugs. In fact, with the advent and development of suitably qualified technical staff within the conventional dispensing process, the pharmacist's role in this area is now steadily reducing and so gives rise to opportunities that make better use of the pharmacist's unique range of skills and expertise alongside those of other members of the healthcare team. Furthermore, the variety and specialisation of the roles performed by pharmacists within different areas of the profession (community, hospital, industry, veterinary, etc.), have also produced considerable variety in what pharmacists actually do in their day-to-day work.

Communication skills (*see Chapter 8*)

The ability to communicate effectively and appropriately is a vital requirement for today's pharmacists. Given the number of people that a pharmacist communicates with on a regular basis – patients and other members of a health-care team (e.g. doctors, dentists, nurses etc.) – it is important that communication is conducted at an appropriate level. For example, consider these two statements:

> If the patient's arterial hypertension is not adequately controlled, there may be a heightened risk of heart attack, stroke, arterial aneurysm or chronic renal failure.

> The medicines you have received are intended to help reduce your high blood pressure. It is very important that you take these medicines in the way the doctor has advised, to keep your blood pressure down. Not taking your medicines is likely to cause your blood pressure to rise, which could eventually lead to increased chances of problems with your heart or kidneys, or of you having a stroke.

It should be obvious that the first statement contains specialised clinical terminology and would be appropriate for a conversation with a doctor, specialist cardiovascular nurse or similar professional clinician; the second statement is more suitable for a conversation with a patient receiving treatment for hypertension. From the examples given above, it should be clear that the way in which pharmacists communicate with the different individuals they encounter in the course of their professional role is critical in getting the right information across in the right way, according to the individual's level of knowledge, need for specific information and relationship to the information being discussed.

Clinical governance (see Chapters 3 & 6)

The term clinical governance describes a systematic approach to maintaining and improving quality of patient care. It has been previously defined as 'A framework through which NHS organisations are accountable for continually improving the quality of their services and safeguarding high standards of care, by creating an environment in which excellence in clinical care will flourish' (Scally & Donaldson, 1998). This definition is based on three key principles:

- recognisably high standards of care
- transparent responsibility and accountability for such standards
- constant improvement.

Standard operating procedures (see Chapters 3 & 12)

Standard operating procedures (SOPs) are an integral part of the pharmacist's role. They comprise detailed written instructions for specific tasks (e.g. dispensing, labelling and checking of medication, disposal of unwanted medicines, etc.) in order to achieve uniformity, safety and efficiency in the performance of the given task. It is critical that SOPs are reviewed regularly (the frequency of review required depends on the nature of the task being described), and also in the event of a near miss or serious incident, all of which require record keeping and review in their own right. The routine use of SOPs and a formalised means of recording, reviewing and reflecting upon (potentially) hazardous incidents enables pharmacists to improve the safety and efficiency of the services they provide to patients.

Adherence, compliance and concordance (Chapter 14)

How patients take their medicine – and whether it is as the prescriber intended – are major issues in ensuring that disease states are treated appropriately. Historically, clinicians took a strongly paternalistic approach to patient care; patients were expected to 'do as they were told' and so to comply and adhere to the prescriber's directions. More recently, this viewpoint has largely fallen into disregard as patients have become much better informed about their own health and the available treatments for the disorders they have. However, one might also argue that, with the advent of the internet and the availability of large amounts of unverified and frequently conflicting information, patients often ultimately end up being less reliably informed! These changes, coupled with broader ranges of information for patients, have resulted in a sea change in patients' and health professionals' perceptions of an effective patient relationship between the patient and health professional.

To this end, a more concordant (concordance: 'a harmony of opinions') approach is now advocated where open discussion between the patient and the health professional(s) involved in his or her care is ongoing, with the aim of agreeing a care plan with the patient that accounts for more than just the prescriber's choice of the best drug. In this regard, factors that might affect a patient's ability or desire to adhere to a treatment plan are considered; these may be issues such as anticipated side-effects, suitable packaging and presentation (what use are child-resistant containers to a patient with chronic arthritis in the hands?), availability (a patient is unlikely to take a medicine that is hard to obtain or unreliable in its supply) and ethical/belief factors (some medicines contain ingredients that may present a dilemma to a patient). Some of these factors, and the influences that they have had on our current concordance-based view and the pharmacist's role in this area are discussed in Chapter 14.

Law and ethics

As with the majority of recognised health professionals, a pharmacist's role is determined by law (e.g. The Medicines Act (1968), The Misuse of Drugs Act (1971)), Royal Pharmaceutical Society of Great Britain (RPSGB) rules and general biomedical ethics. As a result of this, a comprehensive knowledge of the legalities, rules and ethical considerations is a critical requirement for pharmacists; a requirement exemplified by the fact that MPharm students undertake a specific 'Law & Ethics' examination as part of the degree course.

From a pharmacist's point of view, the reasons for this knowledge are twofold.

- Firstly, when acting as gatekeepers in the provision of medicines, they must ensure that they are acting within the constraints laid down in law so as to protect themselves, the patient and the prescriber. A pertinent

example of this is the fact that, at the time of writing, a dispensing error is still considered a criminal offence with which you can be formally charged.
- Secondly, inevitable ethical and legal dilemmas arise frequently during the course of patient care; pharmacists must have a detailed understanding of, and working skills in, the application of ethical principles to guide them through the often difficult choices that they are presented with.

Note that, with the frequent changes to the legal and ethical considerations for pharmacists, any specific and current discussion of law and ethics rapidly becomes out of date. The *MEP* provides up-to-date guidance in this area.

Pharmaceutical care and disease management

The recent and rapidly accelerating change in the pharmacist's role towards more clinical aspects has significantly raised the profile of concepts such as pharmaceutical care, which can be defined as 'the design, implementation, and monitoring of a therapeutic drug plan to produce a specific therapeutic outcome', and disease management – 'the development of integrated treatment plans for patients with long-term conditions'. As can be clearly seen from these definitions, such approaches require considerably more from today's pharmacists than simply dispensing medication in response to a valid prescription, and fully justify an early introduction of Pharmacy Practice within the MPharm degree programme and the more clinical focus of the pharmacist's role.

Clinical interventions (Chapter 15)

A clinical intervention can be defined as 'an action that is intended to alter the course of a disease process or its treatment'. Historically, pharmacists intervened when an error (overdose, inappropriate medication, etc.) was identified on a prescription presented by a patient to a community pharmacy or delivered to the dispensary from a hospital ward. More recently, the increasing clinical focus of the pharmacist's role has broadened the range of situations within which a pharmacist may make an intervention. An understanding of these situations and the ability to deal with them effectively and as part of the larger healthcare team is a critical part of a pharmacist's training.

Continuing professional development (CPD)

The rapid pace of change within the healthcare sector, the introduction of new medications, therapeutic strategies and diagnostic approaches, and the widening role of the pharmacist all mean that every pharmacist must have an ongoing commitment to continuing their own education and training vital for effective performance in their clinical and management roles. To this end, the RPSGB (the representative and regulatory body for pharmacists in the UK (excluding Northern Ireland)) recently introduced a mandatory requirement for annual evidence of accredited demonstration of CPD in order to remain registered as a pharmaceutical chemist. Pharmacists can engage with CPD through a wide variety of routes, including accredited 'on the job' training, distance learning modules (via publications such as the *Pharmaceutical Journal* or *Chemist and Druggist* and online via the Centre for Pharmacy Postgraduate Education (CPPE; www.cppe.manchester.ac.uk)) and events run by the Local Pharmaceutical Committee, to name but a few. The concept of CPD for pharmacy students is frequently introduced early in the MPharm degree programme, often in the form of academic portfolios that encourage reflection on critical events, learning objectives and milestones. Consequently, the majority of today's postgraduate pharmacy students are already familiar with the principles of CPD before registration.

Extemporaneous dispensing *(Chapter 13)*

Extemporaneous dispensing refers to the process of 'freshly' preparing medicines to be provided to a patient, etc. This process, whilst on the wane within the community pharmacy sector, is still a relevant part of the hospital pharmacist's role. As such, a sound ability to extemporaneously prepare medications such as creams, lotions, syrups, suppositories, etc., is still a fundamental requirement for pharmacists. Training and assessment in extemporaneous dispensing skills is an integral part of a pharmacist's (and pharmacy student's) development. As a new area for the majority of students, it can often pose difficulties when adjusting to the conventions, considerations and concerns involved. To address these, this text includes a chapter devoted to specific practical 'tips' for successful extemporaneous dispensing. Extemporaneous dispensing also makes considerable use of a pharmacist's mathematical skills (principally associated with dilutions, concentrations and appropriate mass calculations); thus, competence in this area is an absolute necessity. The reader's attention is drawn to a case in which a pharmacist and pre-registration pharmacy graduate incorrectly prepared Peppermint Water BP for treatment of colic in a baby (*Pharmaceutical Journal*, 2000) because they misunderstood the difference between concentrated chloroform and double-strength chloroform (used in Peppermint Water BP). As a result, too much of this ingredient was used, and the baby died. (See Box 15.10 (page 166) for more details.)

Health psychology and social pharmacy

People experience health and disease in different ways. Each individual's experience is influenced by multiple factors, including their culture, past events, attitudes of family and friends, the society they live in, age, sex, social class, and their understanding of what is happening to them. All these factors will influence how and when patients seek medical help and how they respond to medical (or other health professionals') advice and recommended treatments. In order to help patients gain the most benefit from their treatment, it is essential that pharmacists have an understanding of how these factors may influence a patient's behaviour. This helps pharmacists to adapt their approach to individual patients. In addition, the way in which individual pharmacists (and pharmacy as a profession) are perceived by patients and other health professionals is influenced by social factors. An understanding of these factors can help improve the way pharmacists communicate with these groups and therefore how effectively they practise.

Many of these issues are dealt with throughout this book, particularly patients' experience of health and illness and how this affects medicine taking (Chapter 14).

Drug misuse and its treatment

Drug misuse, whether it presents as a patient's misuse of prescribed/purchased medication or the misuse of illicit drugs such as heroin, cocaine, cannabis, etc., falls within a pharmacist's remit. In the former case, pharmacists are well placed to spot warning signs or indications that a patient may be misusing a medication, such as inappropriate use of a medication that may ultimately lead to the worsening of a condition (e.g. excessive use of 'reliever inhalers' in asthma) or abuse (e.g. of prescribed opioid-based analgesics). In the latter case, pharmacists may encounter illicit drug users when attempts are made to purchase items (e.g. syringes) or chemicals (e.g. citric acid) used in the administration of 'street' drugs. Moreover, if illicit drug users enter sanctioned treatment programmes (e.g. methadone treatment for opioid dependency), their treatments are often dispensed by a single pharmacy and on a daily basis; this treatment and the consumption of the drug can, at the prescriber's discretion, be conducted under the pharmacist's personal supervision.

In both situations, a pharmacist must have a sound appreciation of the associated psychological considerations for the patient, excellent communication skills and a working knowledge of the support systems in place for individuals in such circumstances.

Identification, management and prevention of interactions

In highly simplistic terms, unwanted drug effects can be divided into drug–body interactions (side-effects), drug–drug interactions and drug–food interactions. It should also be borne in mind, however, that the term 'interaction' can be used to describe any effect a drug may have on a patient – including the desired therapeutic effect! Given a pharmacist's expert knowledge of drugs, this is an area where they are very well placed to influence change in a patient's treatment, use of a medication(s), or alterations to diet and lifestyle choices in order to minimise or remove such problems. Other health professionals such as doctors and nurses are often highly reliant on the pharmacist's knowledge in this area in optimising a patient's treatment. The input of the pharmacist is also an invaluable contribution to the concordance-based approach to treatment in which the health professional and patient agree on a treatment plan (described in Chapter 14).

Adverse drug reactions

Adverse drug reactions are dangerous responses in a patient to a particular treatment. We are typically most aware of the risk of adverse reactions with newer drugs, because knowledge about the adverse-effect profile and likely interactions are more limited than with established drugs, and exposure to large patient populations is more limited. However, more established therapies can also produce adverse drug reactions via idiosyncratic effects in some patients.

Moreover, research that uncovers issues associated with new drugs may also raise doubts about established related treatments. For example, the cyclo-oxygenase 2 inhibitors were shown to increase the risk of cardiovascular disease. As a result, further investigation of more established drugs (with a similar mechanism of action) was required to determine whether they pose similar risks. By means of national adverse event reporting systems (e.g. the Yellow Card Scheme for reporting to the Medicines and Healthcare products Regulatory Agency/Committee on Safety of Medicines; see page 27) or local policies, pharmacists are well placed to intervene and to highlight suspected adverse drug reactions by virtue of their expert knowledge.

training received by Pharmacy students and pharmacists, a diverse range of other skills and a competent means of exercising them are vital. Pharmacy Practice lies at the interface of scientific knowledge and these other skills, enabling today's pharmacists to operate effectively, safely and to the benefit of the patient and the healthcare team.

Summary

From this brief overview of some of the main components of Pharmacy Practice it should be clear that, in addition to the extensive scientific

References

Pharm J (2000). 264 (7087): 390–392.

Scally G, Donaldson L J (1998). Clinical governance and the drive for quality improvement in the new NHS in England. *BMJ* 317: 61–65.

2

Structure and function of the NHS in England

Rachel L Howard

Introduction

This chapter describes the structure and function of the National Health Service (NHS) in England. Following devolution of power in the UK, there are significant differences in the structure of the NHS in England, Scotland, Wales and Northern Ireland. Only the NHS in England is described in detail. Different prescription types for each country are, however, described in Chapter 9. This chapter begins by describing the history of the NHS and its structure, followed by recent developments in the NHS. The chapter closes with a description of the roles of pharmacists within the NHS. More detailed information on the roles of pharmacists working within community, hospital and industrial pharmacy is given in Chapters 3, 4 and 5. More detailed information on the history of the NHS and recent changes can be found at www.nhshistory.com.

History of the NHS

In 1942 Sir William Beveridge published *Social Insurance and Allied Services*, a report to the UK government in which he recommended the creation of an NHS to provide care for all citizens through a system of central taxation and other compulsory financial contributions (Beveridge, 1942). In 1946, the National Health Service Act established the structure of the NHS for England and Wales. The NHS was born on 5 July 1948, providing services, free of charge, for the prevention, diagnosis and treatment of disease. This was the first time in the world that completely free health care was made available on the basis of citizenship rather than the payment of fees or insurance premiums (BBC, 1998a).

Before the creation of the NHS in England and Wales, health care was a luxury that usually only the rich could afford. Most hospitals and doctors charged for their care, and many poor people relied on home remedies that could sometimes be dangerous. The creation of an NHS, free at the point of delivery, revolutionised access to health care in England and Wales and contributed to an increase in life expectancy of more than 10 years since 1948. Although no longer truly free (the NHS charges for some services, including prescriptions, spectacles and dental care to some individuals), care provided by general practitioners (GPs) and hospitals remains free at the point of delivery. The NHS largely remains true to its fundamental principles that health care should be free, available to all, and of uniform quality no matter where people live or their background (BBC, 1998b).

Since its creation, the NHS has struggled financially (BBC, 1998a). Demand has always exceeded the resources available, and this has led to repeated changes to the structure of the NHS in an effort to increase efficiency. These changes cycle between centralised management (national policies driving the delivery of health care at a local level) and localised management (local health needs driving the delivery of health care at a local level). The NHS is currently changing from centralised management to localised management (Department of Health, 1997).

Structure of the NHS

The structure of the NHS in England is summarised in Figure 2.1 and is described in more detail below. From a patient's perspective, the NHS is divided into two sectors: primary care and secondary care.

- Primary care is the first point of contact most people have with the NHS. It is delivered by a wide range of health professionals, including GPs, dentists, pharmacists, nurses and opticians. Treatment in primary care focuses on routine injuries and illnesses as well as preventive care (public health), such as helping people to stop smoking. Although primary care is largely responsible for people's general health needs, specialist services are increasingly being provided in primary care to improve access for patients.

- Secondary or acute care is usually provided by an NHS hospital. Services can be provided to patients as outpatients (patients attend hospital services during the day and do not stay overnight) or as inpatients (where patients are admitted to hospital and remain for one or more nights). Admissions to hospital can be planned (elective admissions), for example if a patient needs a non-urgent operation; or unplanned (emergency admissions). More information on services provided by secondary care can be found via the NHS website (ww.nhs.uk).

The Department of Health

The NHS in England is led and supported by the Department of Health (DH) (see Box 2.1), whose remit is 'to improve the health and wellbeing of the people of England' (Department of Health, 2007). The DH is run by six government ministers and over 2000 staff members. The Secretary of State for Health is the senior government minister and overall head of the DH and as such takes overall responsibility for NHS and social care delivery and system reforms, finance and resources, and strategic communications. The Secretary of State for Health, the Prime Minister and other health ministers are advised by the Chief Medical Officer (CMO) (see Box 2.2) on the delivery of health care.

Five further Chief Professional Officers advise the Government and DH on issues relating to nursing, dentistry, health professions, science and pharmacy. The Chief Pharmaceutical Officer (CPO) is the professional lead at the DH responsible for implementing the Pharmacy in the Future programme (see Box 2.3). Further information about the CPO can be found on the Department of Health website (www.dh.gov.uk).

The DH directs national policy on the delivery of health care in England. This policy is given local strategic direction by the strategic health authorities (SHAs) (see Box 2.4). Instead of managing health care directly, the SHAs support the work of local trusts and ensure the quality of that work. Within each SHA the provision of NHS care is divided between different trusts.

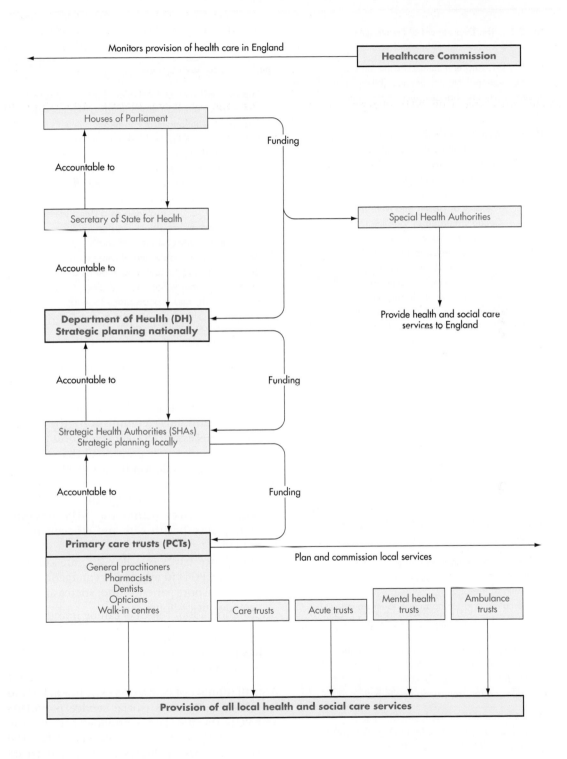

Figure 2.1   Structure of the NHS in England.

Box 2.1   The Department of Health (DH)

The DH sets and communicates the strategic direction for the National Health Service (NHS). The DH has undergone many changes since its creation, as outlined here.

1919	Ministry of Health created to combine the medical and public health functions of central government, and to coordinate/supervise the local health services of England and Wales
1966	Ministry of Health and Ministry of Social Security merged to form the Department of Health and Social Security
1998	Split into the Department of Health and the Department of Social Security
1989	Chief Executive and Leeds-based NHS Executive created in response to the *Working for Patients* White paper.
2003–4	DH reduced in size to six ministers, 2245 staff and three executive agencies

The DH has six key objectives.

1. Improve and protect the health of the population, with special attention to the needs of the poorest, and those with long-term conditions
2. Enhance the quality and safety of services for patients and users
3. Deliver a better experience for patients and users
4. Improve the capacity, capability and efficiency of the health and social care systems
5. Improve the service provided as a department of state to, and on behalf of, ministers and the public, nationally and internationally
6. Become more capable and efficient as a department, and cement reputation as an organisation that is both a good place to do business with, and a good place to work

More information can be found at www.dh.gov.uk/AboutUs/fs/en

Box 2.2   The Chief Medical Officer (CMO)

The first CMO was appointed in 1855 as the principal medical adviser to the government. The CMO is independent of the government, but based at the Department of Health. The CMO's responsibilities include:

1. Preparation of policies and plans, and implementation of programmes to protect the health of the public
2. Promotion and taking action to improve the health of the population and reduce health inequalities
3. Leading initiatives in the National Health Service to enhance quality, safety and standards in clinical services
4. Preparing and reviewing health policy.

More information can be found at www.dh.gov.uk/AboutUs/MinistersAndDepartment Leaders/ChiefMedicalOfficer/fs/en

- Primary care trusts (PCTs) (see Box 2.5) manage and buy (commission) the health services necessary to treat their local population; they are better positioned than SHAs to assess local population health needs.
- NHS acute trusts (see Box 2.6) are commissioned by PCTs to manage the provision of hospital services within the NHS, ensuring high-quality health care and efficient use of money.
- Ambulance trusts (see Box 2.7) are commissioned by PCTs to respond to emergency (999) calls, transport patients, and, increasingly, to provide out-of-hours care.
- Mental health trusts (see Box 2.8) are commissioned by PCTs to provide specialist health and social care for patients with mental health problems.

A small number of care trusts exist in England to help local authorities (social service providers) and PCTs (health service providers) to develop closer working relationships between health and social care. This facilitates a coordinated care package for patients which covers their health

Box 2.3 *Pharmacy in the Future*

Pharmacy in the Future, published by the Department of Health in 2000, set out the role that pharmacists would play in achieving the new NHS plan. It announced a programme of changes to provision of pharmacy services, overseen by the Chief Pharmaceutical Officer. It included three challenges.

1. **Meeting the changing needs of patients** – pharmacists should provide easy access to medicines and advice about medicines, increase support to patients using medicines, and give patients confidence in the advice they receive from pharmacists.
2. **Responding to the changing environment** – community pharmacy is becoming increasingly competitive and patients are demanding novel

services such as electronic ordering and home delivery. Improvements in technology will require further changes to ways of working.

3. **Enhancing public confidence in the profession** – in order to perform expanded services, pharmacists must ensure they are up to date with their knowledge and skills. Continuing professional development must become the norm. Also, arrangements for dealing with things that go wrong must be modernised, for example reporting and learning from errors and near misses.

More information on *Pharmacy in the Future* can be found at the Department of Health website: www.dh.gov.uk

---

Box 2.4 Strategic health authorities (SHAs)

SHAs manage the National Health Service (NHS) locally on behalf of the Secretary of State, and are a key link between the Department of Health and the NHS. SHAs were created in 2000 by merging 100 health authorities. Initially there were 28 SHAs, but these were merged to just 10 in July 2006 to increase efficiency.

SHAs are responsible for:

1. Developing plans to improve health services in their local area
2. Ensuring local health services are high quality and perform well

3. Increasing the capacity of local health services so they can provide more services
4. Making sure national priorities are integrated into local health service plans (e.g. programmes for improving cancer services).

SHAs currently support and monitor the performance of the primary care trusts and hospitals in their geographic area; however, with the creation of the Healthcare Commission (see Box 2.11), the SHAs will become less involved in monitoring performance.

More information on SHAs can be found at www.nhs.uk/England/Aboutnhs

---

Box 2.5 Primary care trusts (PCTs)

PCTs were formed in April 2002 from the primary care groups. Originally, there were 303 PCTs across England, but from October 2006 this number was reduced to 152, to increase efficiency. Most PCTs now share their boundaries with local authorities, in order to better coordinate health and social services.

PCTs report directly to their strategic health authority, and control approximately 80% of the money provided by the Government to spend on health care in England. PCTs manage and pay for local services provided by general practitioners, hospitals, pharmacists, dentists, opticians, mental health services, NHS walk-in centres, NHS Direct, and patient transport.

Box 2.5   Primary care trusts (PCTs) (*continued*)

PCTs are responsible for:

- assessing the health needs of the local population and local community
- commissioning (buying) the right services to meet these needs
- improving the overall health of the local community
- ensuring services can be accessed by everyone who needs them
- listening to, and acting on, patients' views on services
- ensuring that organisations providing services, including social care organisations, work together effectively

- conducting annual assessments of general practices in their area.

Increasingly, PCTs are working with general practices to commission health services (see Box 2.13). Some of the services that PCTs currently provide (e.g. primary care pharmacists, school nurses, etc.) are being removed from direct PCT control as part of a 'commissioner–provider split'. In the future, these services will be commissioned by PCTs and general practice surgeries, and individuals performing these roles will no longer be employed by the PCTs.

Box 2.6   Acute trusts and foundation hospital trusts

Most hospitals within the National Health Service (NHS) are managed by acute trusts. Services provided include: hospital admissions, day surgery (where an overnight stay is not needed) and outpatient services (where patients attend consultations and clinics). Most patients are referred to hospital by their general practitioner (GP) (elective visits), but patients can also attend without a GP referral in emergencies (non-elective or emergency visits).

Acute trusts employ most of the NHS workforce: doctors, nurses, hospital dentists, pharmacists, midwives, health visitors, managers, information technology specialists, physiotherapists, radiographers, podiatrists, speech and language therapists, dietitians, counsellors, occupational therapists, psychologists, and support staff, including receptionists, porters, cleaners, engineers, caterers and domestic and security staff.

Not all hospitals are the same. Some provide specialist centres for disease management. Teaching hospitals are linked to universities and help to train health professionals. Hospitals not linked to universities are usually known as district general hospitals. Hospitals that provide exceptionally efficient and high-quality services can apply to become foundation hospital trusts. These are run by local managers, staff and members of the public. Foundation trust status has many benefits, including greater control over the services provided and less frequent monitoring by the Healthcare Commission (see Box 2.11). Increasingly, some healthcare services traditionally provided by hospitals, such as minor surgery and diagnostic procedures, are being commissioned from independent sector treatment centres – privately run treatment centres which target their services at areas that have traditionally had long waiting times.

---

needs and the social support necessary for a smooth recovery.

In addition to the local trusts, the Government set up special health authorities to provide centralised services to the whole of England (see Box 2.9). NHS Direct was set up under this scheme and, with NHS walk-in centres (see Box 2.10), is commissioned to provide rapid-access health care to the general public.

The provision of health care in England is overseen by the Healthcare Commission, an independent health watchdog (see Box 2.11).

Box 2.7   Ambulance trusts

Thirteen ambulance trusts in England provide emergency services on behalf of primary care trusts (PCTs). Ambulance services are coordinated by a control room, which decides how urgently an ambulance is needed. Levels of urgency are divided into three categories:

A: immediately life-threatening emergencies
B: serious conditions that are not immediately life threatening
C: non-urgent conditions.

The control room decides which service is needed, when to send out a vehicle and which type of vehicle to send – an ambulance or a rapid response vehicle (usually a car) staffed by a paramedic. In non-urgent conditions the control room may recommend contacting the general practitioner or attending a walk-in centre.

In addition to providing emergency transport, many ambulance trusts also provide routine transport for patients to attend hospital clinics.

Box 2.8   Mental health trusts

Although many mental health problems can be treated by general practitioners in primary care, approximately two in every 1000 people will require more specialist care. This care is provided by the mental health trusts. Services include:

* inpatient beds in specialist mental health units
* counselling
* electroconvulsive therapy
* specialist services for children and adolescents
* specialist substance abuse services
* prison mental health services
* mental health crisis resolution
* community-based accommodation
* assessment of offenders for mental health problems
* day care for patients with mental health problems
* assessment, rehabilitation and training in the field of work and employment.

Box 2.9   Special health authorities

Special health authorities provide centralised services to the whole of England. Some of these are described briefly below. Further information on the functions of these authorities can be found on their websites.

* **National Institute for Health and Clinical Excellence** (NICE) makes recommendations on treatments and care using the best available evidence (www.nice.org.uk).
* **National Patient Safety Agency** (NPSA), created in July 2001, coordinates significant event reporting across England, and helps the National Health Service (NHS) to learn from mistakes and problems affecting patient safety (www.npsa.nhs.uk).
* **Health Protection Agency** (HPA) is dedicated to protecting people's health and reducing the impact of infectious diseases, chemical hazards, poisons and radiation hazards (www.hpa.org.uk).
* **National Treatment Agency for Substance Misuse** (NTA) aims to increase the availability, capacity and effectiveness of treatment for drug misuse in England (www.nta.nhs.uk).
* **NHS Blood and Transplant** (NHSBT), created in October 2005, provides a reliable and efficient supply of blood, organs and associated services to the NHS (www.nhsbt.nhs.uk).
* **Information Centre for Health and Social Care** (IC), created in August 2005, collects, analyses and distributes national statistics on health and social care (www.ic.nhs.uk).

Box 2.10   NHS Direct and NHS walk-in centres

NHS Direct was created in March 1998 to provide confidential nurse-led health advice over the telephone 24 hours a day, every day, for example:

- what to do if you or a family member feels ill
- self-care for health conditions such as coughs and colds
- local health services, such as doctors, dentists and out-of-hours pharmacies
- self-help or support organisations.

Additional information for patients is available through the internet (www.nhsdirect.nhs.uk) and the digital television service, including a health encyclopedia and advice on self-management of minor ailments. If patients require non-urgent information, which is not on the website, they can send an enquiry to the information team.

Eighty-four NHS walk-in centres in England provide fast no-appointment advice and treatment for minor conditions. The centres are run by nurses and usually open every day from early morning to late evening. They offer a range of services, including:

- assessment by an experienced National Health Service nurse
- treatment for minor illnesses and injuries
- advice on staying healthy
- information on other health services such as out-of-hours care and dental services.

Further information on NHS Direct and NHS walk-in centres can be found via the NHS website (www.nhs.uk).

Box 2.11   The Healthcare Commission

The Healthcare Commission was created under the Health and Social Care (Community Health and Standards) Act 2003 as an independent health watchdog for England. The Healthcare Commission is accountable to the Secretary of State for Health, and advises and informs the Secretary of State for Health about healthcare provision by, or for, National Health Service (NHS) bodies.

The Healthcare Commission's objectives are:

1. to inspect the quality and value for money of health care and public health

2. to equip patients and the public with the best possible information about healthcare provision
3. to promote improvements in health care and public health.

The Healthcare Commission performs annual checks of each local NHS organisation. Organisations are scored: excellent, good, fair or weak on the basis of the quality of services provided and resource use.

More information can be found at www.healthcarecommission.org.uk.

Recent changes in the NHS

In the 1980s and early 1990s the Conservative government increased the power of GPs in the NHS and introduced performance-related pay by offering financial incentives to encourage improvements in quality of care (Moore *et al.*, 1987). In addition, they created an internal NHS market, arguing that competition between healthcare providers would

also improve the quality of health care. Increasingly, spending power was transferred to primary care (Parliament, 1996a, b). Power in the NHS was centralised, gradually changing 14 regional health authorities into eight regional offices of the DH. Responsibility for planning, funding and delivering health care, however, was split between 100 health authorities, around 3500 GP fundholders (representing half of GP practices) and over 400 NHS acute trusts (Department of Health, 1997).

The New NHS

When the Labour government came to power in 1997, the NHS was once again in financial crisis. This government argued that there was little strategic coordination of NHS services, and that the internal market had increased expenditure on administration, created divisions between health professionals, and led to inequalities in patient care. Labour published *The New NHS. Modern. Dependable* and developed their first 10-year plan to modernise the NHS, replacing the competitive internal market with patient care that would be driven by integration and high standards of performance (Department of Health, 1997). Despite its criticism of the Conservative goverment's changes to the NHS, the majority of Labour's proposed reforms built on these changes, focusing on quality, efficiency and performance, and resulted in the introduction of the National Institute for Clinical Excellence (NICE; now called the National Institute for Health and Clinical Excellence), National Service Frameworks (NSFs), Primary Care Groups (PCGs), the Healthcare Commission and the concept of 'clinical governance' (Rivett, 2007). NICE develops evidence-based guidelines for public health, health technologies and clinical practice (see www.nice.org.uk for more information). The NSFs introduced national standards of care for a range of clinical conditions and patient groups, including older patients and children. Primary care groups (later changed to PCTs) encouraged local GPs and nurses to work together, focusing on prompt, accessible, seamless care delivered to a high standard. The Healthcare Commission was established to ensure high standards of health care throughout the NHS (see Box 2.11).

In addition, proposals to improve NHS performance centred on better use of information technology (Department of Health, 1997). NHS Direct (see Box 2.10) provides 24-hour care via telephone, and the NHSnet and internet allow rapid access to information. Linking laboratories to GPs' computer systems allows results of blood tests to be communicated electronically to GP surgeries, and the National Library for Health (www.library.nhs.uk) provides a wealth of information for health professionals. Patients can also get rapid access to information through NHS Direct online (www.nhsdirect.nhs.uk) and via digital television. Plans still to be implemented include the single electronic patient record. This will be an online record that will provide up-to-date and timely information to health professionals about patients' medical and medication histories, and care they have received.

The NHS Plan

The changes in healthcare provision set out in *The New NHS. Modern. Dependable* (Department of Health, 1997) did not achieve what the Labour government hoped for. Therefore, in their second term in government, Labour announced further changes, with the publication of their second 10-year plan 'The NHS Plan' (Department of Health, 2000a). These changes encompassed government spending on the NHS (to increase by 50% over 5 years), staffing, infrastructure and patient involvement in the NHS. As a result of these changes, patients:

- can influence how NHS services are organised through patient consultations and patient advisory and liaison services (PALS) (where patients can comment on the health care they have received and suggest changes)
- receive more information about the type of care they receive and the performance of hospitals where they receive care
- choose which local provider they want to receive their care from.

Staffing changes included:

- increased numbers of, and better paid, healthcare staff – numbers of health professionals were initially increased under the Labour reforms; however, financial difficulties, caused by underestimating the cost of new contracts for doctors (under the new GP and consultant contracts) and other staff (under Agenda for Change) have meant that staffing levels are falling again

- new contracts of employment for hospital consultants (October 2003) and GPs (April 2004) – the new GP contract included payments through the Quality and Outcomes Framework (QOF) (see Box 2.12), which has acted as an incentive for GPs to improve services to patients
- better use of healthcare staff skills – the roles of many non-medical health professionals have been extended. For example, appropriately qualified pharmacists and nurses can now prescribe medicines within the confines of a clinical management plan which is agreed with the patient and doctor (supplementary prescribing) or independently (independent prescribers).

Changes to NHS infrastructure included:

- building new hospitals and GP surgeries
- increased training places for medical students
- creation of foundation trusts for hospitals that perform exceptionally well
- creation of care trusts to facilitate closer working between healthcare and social care providers
- closer working with private providers of health care – local commissioning of health-

care services now allows private providers to perform minor surgery for example. The private sector is increasingly becoming an integral part of NHS care.

Shifting the balance of power

In 2001, the Secretary of State for Health announced further changes to the NHS in a series of speeches and white papers called '*Shifting the balance of power*', in order to achieve the objectives set out in the *NHS Plan* (Department of Health, 2001a, b; 2002). These changes included:

- shifting commissioning of healthcare services to PCTs
- devolving responsibility for the strategic direction of local healthcare services to SHAs (Box 2.4).

Creating a patient-led NHS

In 2005, further guidance on implementing the *NHS Plan* was announced through the '*Creating a Patient-led NHS*' programme (Department of Health, 2005). This consisted of a series of white papers detailing how patients should become more involved in decisions about the

---

Box 2.12   Quality and Outcomes Framework (QOF)

The QOF forms part of the General Medical Services contract introduced in April 2004. It provides financial incentives to general practitioners to encourage provision of high-quality care. The QOF measures the achievement of general practices against a range of evidence-based clinical, practice organisation, and management indicators. Practices score points according to their levels of achievement against these indicators, and payments to practices are calculated from the points achieved. These payments can then be used to further improve patient care. The QOF is divided into four domains:

- **clinical** – 76 indicators in 11 disease areas, including heart disease, lung disease, diabetes and epilepsy. The majority of points are awarded in this domain

- **organisational** – 56 indicators in five areas including record keeping, communication with patients, and medicines management
- **patient experience** – four indicators covering patient survey and consultation length
- **additional services** – ten indicators in four areas, including cervical screening, child health surveillance, maternity services and contraceptive services.

The indicators are reviewed each year to encourage further improvements in quality of care.

Further information on the QOF can be found at www.ic.nhs.uk/services/qof and www.primarycarecontracting.nhs.uk.

provision of healthcare services, and health professionals in the commissioning of local healthcare services through practice-based commissioning (see Box 2.13). It was hoped that increased patient control over the provision of health services would improve cost effectiveness and efficiency in the NHS (Wanless, 2002). In addition, the introduction of 'payment by results' (see Box 2.14) was also intended to increase efficiency. These reports also paved the way for reducing the number of SHAs from 28 to 10 and PCTs from 303 to 152, in order to create more money to spend directly on patient care by reducing the money spent on management. In addition, these changes meant that many PCTs have the same boundaries as local authorities, making it easier to link the provision of health care and social care.

Pharmacist roles within the NHS

Of all the health professionals, pharmacists have the most detailed education in the use of medicines. They are ideally placed to support other health professionals in medicines management and, increasingly, to take the lead in managing patients. This potential was recognised in *'Pharmacy in the Future: Implementing the NHS Plan'* (see Box 2.3) (Department of Health, 2000b). Pharmacists mostly work within three areas of the NHS: community pharmacies, hospitals and primary care. Further information on the roles of pharmacists working in different areas is available in a series of articles published in the *Pharmaceutical Journal* (available via www.pharmj.com) and in Chapters 3 and 4.

Box 2.13   Practice-based commissioning (PBC)

PBC is an opportunity for all primary health professionals (not just GPs) to improve services for their local populations. Practices can work with their local primary care trusts (PCTs) to commission these services. Practices decide which services are needed, whilst PCTs manage the bureaucracy of commissioning services and provide incentives to engage practices in the commissioning process. Many PCTs are recommending that practices form clusters (groups of practices with similar patient groups) for commissioning because larger groups will have more power to buy the services they need. Practices are encouraged to think creatively about new ways to provide services. It is hoped that PBC will transfer some services from secondary care to primary care, making such services more accessible to patients and more cost efficient. Practices will be allowed to keep up to 70% of the cost savings generated by PBC to further improve patient care locally.

More information about PBC can be found on the Department of Health website (www.dh.gov.uk).

Box 2.14   Payment by results (PbR)

PbR aims to provide a transparent, rules-based system for paying hospitals for the services they provide. In the past, hospitals were paid in advance for their services through 'block contracts'. Contracts were negotiated locally and the amount paid was based on the expected workloads. If less work than expected was done, hospitals kept the extra money; if more was done than expected, hospitals were paid for the extra work. PbR moves away from this system by paying a fixed rate (tariff) for a service each time it is provided. The tariff is calculated from the average cost of providing a service. If a service is provided for less than the tariff cost, then the provider will make a profit. Conversely, if the service costs more than the tariff, the provider will make a loss. This will encourage efficiency.

More information on PbR can be found on the Department of Health website (www.dh.gov.uk).

Community pharmacists

The majority of pharmacists (70%) work in community pharmacy (Hassell *et al.*, 2006) and 80% of their work is for the NHS (Department of Health, 2003b). The major work of community pharmacists involves supplying medicines to the public, either by dispensing prescriptions or by selling medicines to treat minor ailments. A community pharmacist must be present at a pharmacy for medicines to be supplied. The supply of medicines requires pharmacists to perform a number of tasks, including:

- assessing the safety of prescriptions for patients
- ensuring that prescriptions and medication labels are legal and accurate
- advising patients on how and when to take their medicines, which medicines to avoid, and possible side-effects of medicines and what to do if they occur
- advising patients which over-the-counter medicine they should take to treat a minor ailment.

Increasingly, the community pharmacist's role is expanding into new and exciting areas, helped by the introduction of the new Pharmacy Contract, extension of prescribing rights to non-medical health professionals, and support by the general public (Department of Health and HM Government, 2006). The changes to the NHS described earlier have opened up new opportunities for community pharmacists (Department of Health, 2003b). PCTs and general practices are now commissioning community pharmacists to provide services that would only previously have been supplied by hospitals or GPs (Primary Care Contracting, 2006).

- **Medicines use reviews** – community pharmacists are paid to liaise with patients about their medicines. Community pharmacists have the opportunity to assess patient understanding, identify problems and provide solutions. Another medicines management role is visiting patients at home after discharge from hospital, helping them to avoid problems with their medication such as confusion over which medicines to take, difficulties opening packaging or side-effects from medication.

- **Minor ailments schemes** – community pharmacists can supply medicines free of charge to patients (who would not normally pay for their medicines) to help treat minor ailments such as fever, cough, etc. Such schemes reduce the need for patients to attend hospital emergency departments.
- **Public health schemes** – some community pharmacies offer smoking cessation clinics and help with obesity management (Department of Health, 2003a).
- **Substance misuse support** – community pharmacists can provide needle exchange schemes, observed methadone administration and other support services to help drug addicts or misusers of other substances to stop.
- **Point of care testing** – community pharmacies can offer testing for disease management (e.g. for diabetes, heart disease or anticoagulation monitoring). These services can also involve diagnostic testing for heart disease or diabetes. These services help the NHS to meet the standards set out in the NSFs.
- **Repeat dispensing** – patients receive repeat supplies of their medication without needing to contact their GP surgery. This differs from repeat prescribing, where a patient requests a signed prescription from the GP surgery and then takes it to the pharmacy.
- **Patient education** – in addition to counselling patients about their medication, community pharmacists can also run education sessions about general disease management, and provide written information on a range of conditions, medicines and services.

In addition, community pharmacists are often responsible for managing their businesses, and must therefore run the pharmacy efficiently and profitably. This can include financial management (ensuring that the pharmacy makes a profit), merchandising (advertising the products sold in the pharmacy), responsibility for staff and premises (people management), stock control (ensuring that sufficient stock is available to meet customer demands), stock rotation (ensuring that old stock is used before new stock) and ordering. To keep their pharmacies profitable, pharmacists often sell non-pharmaceutical products such as cosmetics, toiletries and photographic products (including developing and printing photos).

During their working day, community pharmacists work closely with patients (advising them on their medicines) and prescribers (helping them select the most appropriate medication for a patient or resolving problems with prescriptions). They also work closely with pharmacy support staff such as technicians and counter assistants. Further information on the role of community pharmacists is given in Chapter 3.

Hospital pharmacists

Around 20–25% of pharmacists work in hospital pharmacies (Hassell *et al.,* 2006), performing essential roles in medicines' supply and ensuring that medicines are used safely, effectively and economically (Audit Commission, 2001; Department of Health, 2003b). This complex role involves working closely with patients, doctors, nurses, other health professionals, and pharmacy support staff (technicians and assistant technical officers). Pharmacists perform numerous roles in the hospital setting:

- checking hospital prescription charts for legibility, accuracy, legality and clinical appropriateness, in the dispensary and on the ward
- overseeing the dispensing of medicines to hospital wards and patients
- clarifying patients' medication histories on admission to hospital
- organising patients' medication for discharge from hospital
- discussing patients' medication regimens with them, ensuring they understand when and how to take the medications, what to take them for and important side-effects to look for and what to do if they occur
- liaising with doctors to ensure that prescriptions are clinically appropriate and cost-effective
- liaising with nursing staff to ensure that medicines are stored and administered appropriately
- answering enquiries from health professionals and the public about medicines

- organising supplies of medicines for use in clinical trials.

As the focus of the NHS has turned to efficiency and quality, hospital pharmacists must respond by providing efficient and safe supply of medicines as part of the drive to increase the efficiency and quality of care in the hospitals they work for. In common with community pharmacists, the role of hospital pharmacists has expanded with the changes in the NHS. Pharmacists are increasingly taking part in ward rounds, prescribing medicines as supplementary or independent prescribers (or under the direction of hospital consultants as part of a patient group direction), promoting the appropriate and rational use of antibiotics, overseeing the production of specialised products not available from pharmaceutical companies, and helping to ensure that patients are safely discharged by liaising with community and primary care pharmacists.

Further information on the roles of hospital pharmacists in the NHS can be found in a series of careers articles published in *Hospital Pharmacist* (available from www.pharmj.com/hp) and in Chapter 4.

Primary care pharmacists

Only 8% of pharmacists work in primary care, the newest role for pharmacists (Hassell *et al.,* 2006). Primary care pharmacists are taking on new roles and working in new areas where pharmacists have not traditionally been present, such as general practices. Pharmaceutical advisers have strategic roles, directing the provision of services and overseeing the use of medicines in their local area. Practice pharmacists have clinical roles similar to that of hospital pharmacists. They work closely with patients and GPs to ensure safe and cost-effective use of medicines. Primary care pharmacists can help general practices to reduce the amount of money spent on medicines by switching to cheaper equally effective products, where appropriate, and to develop formularies. They help general practices to adhere to guidelines for medicines' usage developed by NICE and to meet targets for medicines' management detailed in the NSFs and QOF. Primary care pharmacists support GPs in reducing inappropriate prescribing that might otherwise contribute to hospital admissions. They reduce GP workloads by conducting medicine review clinics and reviewing hospital discharge prescriptions (the medicines that patients are prescribed when they leave hospital), helping to ensure that patients are treated optimally when they return home.

Summary

This chapter should have given you a better understanding of the structure of the NHS and how recent changes have affected healthcare provision in England. In addition, you should have an appreciation of the rapidly expanding roles of pharmacists in healthcare provision.

References

Audit Commission (2001). *A Spoonful of Sugar – Medicines Management in NHS Hospitals*, London: Audit Commission. (Accessible via www.audit-commission.gov.uk.)

BBC (1998a). The NHS: 'One of the greatest achievements in history'. Available from http://news.bbc.co.uk/1/hi/events/nhs_at_50/special_report/ 123511.stm (accessed 23 January 2007).

BBC (1998b). True to its principles? Available from http://news.bbc.co.uk/1/hi/events/nhs_at_50/special_report/125891.stm (23 January 2007).

Beveridge W (1942). *Social Insurance and Allied Services (The Beveridge Report)*. CMND 6404, London: Stationery Office.

Department of Health (1997) *The New NHS. Modern. Dependable*. Cm 3807.

Department of Health (2000a). *The NHS Plan: a Plan for Investment, a Plan for Reform*. London: Stationery Office.

Department of Health (2000b). *Pharmacy in the Future: Implementing the NHS Plan*. London: Department of Health.

Department of Health (2001a). *Shifting the Balance of Power Within the NHS: Securing Delivery*. London: Department of Health.

Department of Health (2001b). *Shifting the Balance of Power: Securing Delivery – Human Resources Framework*. London: Department of Health.

Department of Health (2002). *Shifting the Balance of Power: the Next Steps*. London: Department of Health.

Department of Health (2003a).*Tackling Health Inequalities: A Programme for Action*. London: Department of Health.

Department of Health (2003b). *A Vision for Pharmacy in the New NHS*. London: Department of Health.

Department of Health (2005). *Creating a Patient-led NHS: Delivering the NHS Improvement Plan*. London: Department of Health.

Department of Health (2007). Department of Health: *About Us*. Available from http://www.dh.gov.uk/AboutUs/fs/en (accessed 25 January 2007).

Department of Health & HM Government (2006). *Our Health, Our Care, Our Say: a New Direction for Community Services*. Cm 6737, London: Stationery Office.

Hassell K, Seston L, Eden M (2006). *Pharmacy Workforce Census 2005: Main Findings*. University of Manchester.

Moore J, Walker P, King T, Rifkind M (1987) *Promoting Better health: the Government's Programme for Improving Primary Health Care*. Cm 249, London: Stationery Office.

Parliament (1996a). *Choice and Opportunity. Primary Care: the Future*. Cm 3390, London: Stationery Office.

Parliament (1996b) *Primary Care: Delivering the Future*. Cm 3512, London: Stationery Office.

Primary Care Contracting (2006). *Practice Based Commissioning (PBC) Bulletin 5 – Pharmacy and PBC*. Available from www.primarycarecontracting.nhs.uk (accessed 30 January 2007).

Rivett G (2007). *Introduction to the Decade from 1998*. Available from www.nhshistory.net (accessed 30 January 2007).

Wanless D (2002). *Securing Our Future Health: Taking A Long-Term View. Final Report*. London: HM Treasury.

3

An overview of community pharmacy – the role of the community pharmacist: past, present and future

Sam E Weston

Introduction

More pharmacists currently work in the community sector than in any other part of the pharmaceutical industry – nearly 75% work in this setting, either employed by multiple pharmacy chains as pharmacists, pharmacy or store managers or relief pharmacists, or self-employed as pharmacy owners or locums. This role has changed significantly over the years, and continues to develop at a rapid pace as pharmacists rise to the challenges and changes presented to them by the ever-changing National Health Service (NHS).

In the UK, a community pharmacist can expect to consult with up to 15 patients a day on an over-the-counter (OTC) basis (Figure 3.1), as well as interacting with patients who are presenting prescription forms or collecting dispensed medications. At the time of writing, a community pharmacist rarely has access to a patient's full confidential medical record,

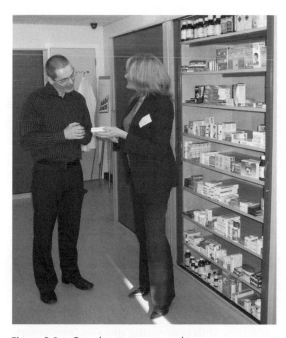

Figure 3.1 Over-the-counter prescribing.

although many strategic health authorities are seeking to improve this and are looking at ways to introduce electronic access for pharmacists. The current lack of access means that pharmacists must rely heavily on their communication skills to obtain relevant information from a patient to allow for correct diagnosis and supply of treatment – or referral to a general practitioner (GP) if appropriate.

This chapter provides an overview of the changes in the role of the community pharmacist, the current situation and possible future developments of services provided by community pharmacists.

The past role of the community pharmacist

Wherever there are civilised societies we find pharmacy, because it fulfils one of man's basic needs – the maintenance of health. The development of medicines from plants, animals and insects became routine thousands of years ago, long before it became a part of the profession we now recognise. However, we must not forget that the same skills and knowledge that bring healing and health can also be used to destroy – inappropriate dosing of medication, potential interactions or medicines that are simply unsuitable for a certain patient should be identified by the pharmacist. In addition to this, the quality of advice and information provided to the patient by the pharmacist, or by supporting healthcare staff, should be monitored in order to ensure that patients receive the best possible care. In the event that such procedures are not carried out, it is possible that medications prescribed or advice given to patients may cause them harm rather than benefit their health. Pharmacists today are ideally placed in the front line of health care. Within the domain of the general public and armed with a huge knowledge of medicines and poisons, they are able to identify existing disease states and offer suitable treatment. In addition, they can supply advice and information for the prophylactic use of medicines, thus preventing diseases from arising in the first place.

Pharmacy has a long history. Fossils from plants with medicinal properties have been found with the remains of Neanderthals, indicating that early man used these plants as drugs around 50 000 BC. The first prescription of which we have authentic records is now in the British Museum and dates back to 3700 BC, although it is not confirmed whether this script was found in the tomb of a patient or whether it was recovered from the effects of a pharmacist. The earliest historical record for the preparation of drugs comes from Babylonia, circa 2600 BC, where clay tablets were inscribed with the description of an illness, a formula for the preparation of the remedy and an incantation to impart or enhance the healing quality of the medication.

A more detailed history of pharmacy dates back to medieval times. when priests, both men and women, ministered to the sick with religious rites as well as medicines. Specialisation first occurred early in the 9th century in the civilised world around Baghdad, where the first privately owned drug stores were established. It gradually spread to Europe as alchemy, eventually evolving into chemistry as physicians began to abandon beliefs that were not demonstrable in the physical world. Physicians often both prepared and prescribed medicines (comparable with today's dispensing doctors), whilst pharmacists not only compounded prescriptions but also manufactured medicaments in bulk for general sale (see Figures 3.2–3.5). Not until well into the 19th century was the distinction between the pharmacist as a specialist in the preparation of medicines and the physician as a therapist generally accepted.

Combining different agents, or compounding, was considered an art form practised by priests and doctors and the first known chemical processes were carried out by the artisans of Mesopotamia, Egypt and China. Most of these craftspeople were employed in temples and palaces, making luxury goods for priests and nobles. In the temples, the priests in particular had time to speculate on the origin of the changes they saw in the world about them. Their theories often involved what was perceived as magic, but they also developed astronomical, mathematical and cosmological

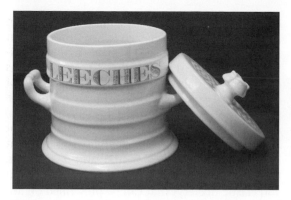

Figure 3.2 A leech jar, used to store leeches. Blood letting was a universal practice in ancient Greek and Roman times. By the 1700s, apothecaries and physicians used leeches instead of opening a vein. They were also used to treat infected wounds and to promote healing of tissues.

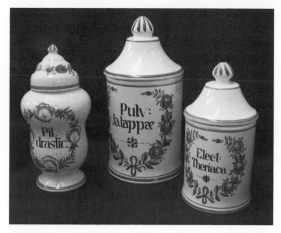

Figure 3.4 Storage jars for dried herbs used in the preparation of 'pills'.

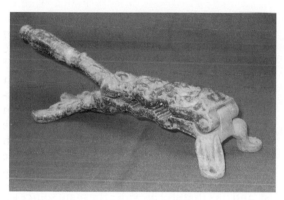

Figure 3.3 A press used for making suppositories (for rectal administration of medicines) or pessaries (for vaginal administration).

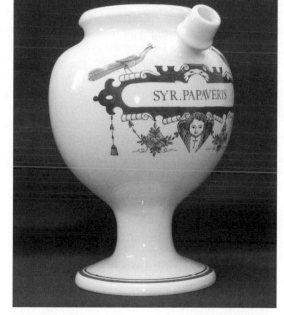

Figure 3.5 A syrup jar used to store *Syrupus Papaveris* – an analgesic and anti-inflammatory medicine prepared by infusing dried poppy heads and seeds in boiling water and sugar.

ideas, which they then used in attempts to explain some of the changes that are now considered chemical (British Society for the History of Pharmacy, 2007). More information can be found on the British Society for the History of Pharmacy website (www.bshp.org).

Pharmacy first became legally separated from medicine in 1231 AD in Sicily and southern Italy. King Frederick of Sicily, Emperor of Germany, presented the first European edict differentiating between the responsibilities of physicians and apothecaries at his palace in Palermo. This paved the way for further legislation defining

the role of apothecary, the development of the first official pharmacopoeia (the *Ricettario Florentino* published in Florence in 1498), the establishment of the College de Pharmacie in France in 1777 and the eventual formation of the Pharmaceutical Society of Great Britain in 1841 (Taylor & Harding, 2001).

During the 19th century, the art of compounding began to give way to new technologies. However, it has been estimated that a 'broad knowledge of compounding' was still essential for 80% of the prescriptions dispensed in the 1920s. Although pharmacists increasingly relied on chemicals purchased from the manufacturer to make up prescriptions, there still remained much to be done *secundum artem* ('to make favourably with skill') at the time of preparation and dispensing. Pharmacists spread their own plasters, prepared pills (of aloes and myrrh or quinine and opium, for example), prepared powders of all kinds, and made up confections, conserves, medicated waters and perfumes. They also prepared tinctures (of, for example, laudanum, paregoric and colchicum) in five-gallon demijohns. Frequently, pharmacists combined into a single dosage form (a 'pill'), two or more medicines, which would today be written and dispensed as separate items on a prescription. This allowed them to take advantage of what were considered to be favourable interactions between medicines, or simply to reduce the number of pills taken by a patient, thus improving the chance of the patient taking medications correctly. Pharmacists were often called upon to provide first aid and medicines for such common ailments as burns, frostbite, colic, flesh wounds, poisoning, constipation and diarrhoea, as a consultation with a physician for such minor ailments was costly. Pharmacists then, as today, were a first-line of defence in these situations, as they could provide advice and supply a treatment at the same time and for a much reduced price.

In addition to maintaining a prescription laboratory, pharmacists usually carried patented and proprietary remedies along with herbs and locally popular *nostrums* ('a favourite but untested remedy for problems or evils') of their own design.

Today, the modern pharmacist deals with complex pharmaceutical remedies far different from the elixirs, spirits and powders described in the *Pharmacopoeia of London* (1618) and the *Pharmacopoeia of Paris* (1639). In the UK today, major medicines are selected for inclusion in the *British Pharmacopoeia* (*BP*), first published in English (previously in Latin) in 1864. These medicinal substances are required to reach rigorously tested standards before being considered for inclusion. Once produced as medicinal products, medicines are listed in the bi-annually updated *British National Formulary* (*BNF*), a compendium of all medicines and appliances (such as catheters, wound-management products and elastic hosiery) that can be prescribed on an NHS prescription form. The *BNF* also provides guidance about medications that cannot be prescribed on an NHS prescription – known as 'blacklisted' medicines – and medicines that are considered less suitable for prescribing.

Today's community pharmacist

Pharmacists are experts in the use of medicines. They complete a 3 year masters degree and a year of practical training, and must pass an examination before qualifying to register with the Royal Pharmaceutical Society of Great Britain (RPSGB) as a Pharmaceutical Chemist (Parliamentary Office of Science and Technology, 2005).

The traditional role of the community pharmacist, and one that still provides the main source of income for the majority of pharmacies, is that of dispensing. In 2005, 720 million prescription items were dispensed (Figure 3.6), an increase of 5% from 2004 (IC, 2006). The largest growth area in terms of volume is cardiovascular disease, in terms of both prescription items dispensed and net ingredient cost. Other disease states that place a high cost burden on the NHS include diabetes, gastrointestinal disorders and respiratory diseases (IC, 2007).

Other roles of the community pharmacist are largely divided into two categories:

- essential services – provided by virtually every pharmacy in the UK
- enhanced services – developed in line with the new NHS contract discussed in Chapter 2.

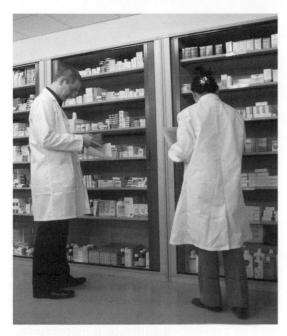

Figure 3.6   A working dispensary.

Essential services

Repeat dispensing

A community pharmacist can supply medication to the patient in the event that the patient receives a regular prescription from their GP for a particular condition, has been maintained successfully without need for any change to the medication regimen for a period of time, and is not due for a GP review of their medications. GPs supply prescriptions in advance to the pharmacy, allowing a reduction in their workload, as well as reduced drug wastage and greater use of the pharmacist's skills.

Adverse drug reaction reporting

The Yellow Card Scheme was launched in 1964, and is used to report suspected adverse drug reactions (ADRs) to the Medicines and Health-care products Regulatory Authority (MHRA) and Committee on Safety of Medicines (CSM). Both

hard copies (the yellow pages in the back of the BNF) and electronic versions (implemented in 2002 and available at www.mhra.gov.uk) of the yellow card are currently in use. Reports are divided into two categories:

- 'black triangle drugs' (noted as such in the BNF; these are drugs that have received market authorisation in the last 2 years) for which any suspected ADRs should be reported
- all other drugs, for which only serious suspected ADRs should be reported.

Currently the Yellow Card Scheme can be used by doctors, nurses, pharmacists, dentists, coroners, optometrists and radiographers (www.mhra.gov.uk). Members of the public are now able to use this scheme, both online and by directly contacting the manufacturer of a medication that may have caused an adverse event. This has allowed for more comprehensive profiles to be developed for any medicine that may have caused a suspected adverse reaction. More information about the Yellow Card Scheme can be found on the MHRA website (www.mhra.gov.uk).

Patient counselling

This involves giving advice to patients on how to use their prescribed medications, often used as an informal method of checking on how patients are coping with their medications. Early identification of problems, such as timing of medications, side-effects or problems with physical manipulation of the packaging can be addressed promptly, with minimum disruption to the patient's lifestyle.

Identification of interactions of prescribed medications with other medicines, herbal remedies and foodstuffs

The ageing population, both in the UK and worldwide (United Nations, 2001) means that many more patients are taking more than one clinically justified medication – so-called polypharmacy – thus increasing the potential for drug–drug interactions.

The re-emergence of herbal supplements as beneficial to health, as well as their increasing popularity as complementary medicines, leads to another host of possible interactions. Many people hold firmly to the misconception that 'natural is good', which suggests, incorrectly, that herbal medicines have none of the side-effects or toxicity problems that arise with 'unnatural' medicines.

New research has shown that some foods have enzyme inhibiting or enhancing effects (such as grapefruit juice). The community pharmacist is ideally placed to question patients about potential interactions and to counsel patients before such interactions occur.

Responding to symptoms

Community pharmacists can provide advice on appropriate purchase of OTC and pharmacy (P) medicines (which can only be sold under the supervision of a pharmacist) for symptomatic relief in the case of self-limiting minor illnesses and common complaints. In this situation the community pharmacist needs to draw on an extensive group of skills:

- communication skills in order to draw out relevant information from the patient, as well as to impart health advice
- clinical skills in order to interpret symptoms and determine a therapeutic objective
- knowledge of current OTC medication in order to recommend a suitable product
- directing the patient to their GP in the event that symptoms may suggest a more serious complaint.

Public health

This involves participation in local and national campaigns to raise awareness of specific health issues. Promotions (organised both centrally and locally) include smoking cessation clinics, raising awareness of the risk factors that contribute to major disease states such as heart disease (e.g. improving diet and exercise regimens), diabetes (e.g. monitoring blood glucose levels), promoting influenza vaccination for at-risk patients (the elderly and those with chronic respiratory diseases) and advice on appropriate use of antibiotics. The prescribing of antibiotics for the treatment of viral infections is inappropriate and is one factor that is contributing to the growing problem of antibiotic-resistance in bacteria. Antibiotic resistance can also occur if patients do not take a course of antibiotics correctly – the bacteria that the medicine is supposed to kill can develop resistance to it and then, in the event that the patient requires the antibiotic to treat another bacterial infection, a higher dose may be required, or the antibiotic may not prove effective, because the bacteria have become resistant to it. Pharmacists occupy a valuable position in this regard by being able to intervene at the point of dispensing if they feel that a prescribed antibiotic is inappropriate.

Signposting

Referral of patients to the most appropriate healthcare providers in order to reduce inappropriate use of health and social care services (e.g. frequent visits from GPs, practice nurses, physiotherapists). Lists are provided by primary care trusts (PCTs), and include voluntary patient support groups. Often patients can get advice from telephone help lines such as NHS Direct or from the internet (e.g. www.nhsdirect.nhs.uk).

Disposal of unwanted medications

The aims of this service are:

- to reduce the incidence of accidental poisoning in the home, and the risk of medications being diverted to individuals they were not intended for
- to reduce the risk to the public caused by medicines disposed of unsafely
- to reduce the environmental impact of unsafe disposal.

Patients are requested to return unused medicines to the community pharmacy for safe disposal in destruction of old pharmaceuticals (DOOP) bins, which are then collected by a pharmaceutical waste disposal company (contracted by the PCT).

Clinical governance

Clinical governance refers to 'a framework through which NHS organisations are accountable for continuously improving the quality of their services and safeguarding high standards of care, by creating an environment in which excellence in clinical care will flourish' (National Prescribing Centre, 2007). This is a large area that affects every aspect of the pharmacist's role and is characterised by:

- audit – defined as an important review of current practice, revision of any part of practice which does not give the best standards of care for patients, and integration of new procedures for improving these standards
- continuing professional development
- accreditation training
- staff development programmes
- development and implications of standard operating procedures (SOPs)

within the community pharmacy setting (see Chapters 6 and 15).

Medicines use review (MUR)

This is an advanced service that requires both pharmacist and premises to be accredited from a higher education institution (e.g. The Centre for Inter-Professional Postgraduate Education and Training (CIPPET; www.pharmacy.rdg.ac.uk/cippet) or the Centre for Pharmacy Postgraduate Education (CPPE; www.cppe.manchester.ac.uk). MURs can be routine (when a pharmacist and patient make an appointment to meet and discuss the patient's treatment regimen, and address any issues, such as side-effects or unused medications being stopped on a regular prescription), or may be triggered by prescription intervention (such as when a pharmacist notices a potential interaction or that a patient may be receiving a new drug in order to counter side-

effects produced by a regular medication). An MUR involves a face-to-face consultation with the patient in order to examine current medicine usage, check for potential side-effects and produce a report, which is copied to the patient's GP, suggesting changes in the medication schedule if necessary. Specific patient groups to be routinely included in the MUR protocol for a pharmacy may be suggested by PCTs depending on the needs of a particular area (e.g. patients over 70 years of age; patients with hypertension; patients with diabetes).

Other services

Retailing

Most community pharmacists are also business people. Those employed as managers and those who are pharmacy owners have an obvious requirement to run the pharmacy as a profit-making organisation. In addition, the pharmacist must have managerial skills in order to direct and develop their support staff, as well being involved in reviewing the needs and requirements of the patients who use their premises. Managers need to develop skills in many areas:

- strategic planning – both for the business as a whole, and for individual members of staff
- financial strategy and planning – an essential component for running any business successfully, both for review of past performance and also for future budget plans
- problem solving – often managers are required to think 'outside the box' and come up with a highly creative solution to a problem that can be enthusiastically taken on board by staff members
- marketing – the right advertising is needed in order to attract the right support staff and also to bring in customers.

Locally enhanced services

These are commissioned by PCTs, in response to local healthcare needs and so will vary from one

PCT area to another. Community pharmacies do not have to provide all of these services, but the PCT area will ensure that all the required services are catered for between the community pharmacies in one healthcare authority. They include the following services.

Smoking cessation clinics

These clinics have been developed in order to reduce the number of minor consultations with GPs, helping to reduce their workloads. An initial screening is often done by a practice nurse before the patient is referred to a community pharmacist. The pharmacist can then assess the needs of the patient and carry out peak flow measurements, which are a useful measure for the patient to see how their lung function improves the longer they do not smoke.

Minor ailments schemes

These were also created in order to reduce minor consultations for GPs in order to free up their time to treat more seriously ill patients, as well as to utilise more effectively the medicines knowledge of qualified and registered pharmacists. Patients can be prescribed antihistamines and steroid nasal sprays for hay fever, decongestants and analgesics for cold and flu symptoms, and pain relief, cough mixtures, etc. In this way patients are provided with symptomatic relief from a minor ailment, without a perhaps unnecessary visit to the GP, which can also be time-consuming for the patient; indeed they may have recovered from the illness by the time they get to see the doctor.

Substance misuse

Patients with a drug dependency (e.g. heroin, amphetamines or painkillers) can be started on a programme of withdrawal. Specialist GPs or substance misuse clinics can supply prescriptions for methadone (a drug that prevents the onset of withdrawal symptoms experienced by users of opioids such as heroin), which can be supplied as a single dose on a daily basis (either as supervised consumption on the pharmacy premises, or to take away) or as a week's supply

of daily doses. The community pharmacist is ideally situated to monitor these patients' progress and to provide continuing support.

Emergency hormonal contraception

The 'morning-after pill' to prevent unwanted pregnancy has been available from GPs and family planning clinics for many years. Community pharmacies are now allowed to sell this product as a 'P' licensed product, or to supply it free of charge if a patient group directive (PGD) is in existence in their PCT (Department of Health, 2007). Pharmacists must undergo training to be able to prescribe on a PGD form. This is a document that makes it legal for medicines to be given to a defined group of patients by suitably trained health professionals other than a doctor, without an individual prescription having to be written for each patient.

Advice to residential and care homes

Community pharmacies can supply residential homes with medication in weekly dispensing trays and monitored dosage systems. This helps to ensure that patients receive their medication at the correct time, and improves the ease of administration for home staff. Community pharmacists are often closely involved with reviewing these medications and provide advice to home staff and carers in order to provide the highest standard of care for the patient group. Further details of training requirements for pharmacists and technicians for the 'Home away from home' programme can be found on the CPPE website (www.cppe.manchester.ac.uk).

Health screening

Services for monitoring blood cholesterol, blood sugar and blood pressure are now routinely provided in the majority of community pharmacies, as many patients are beginning to take a more active role in understanding and treating their illness (RPSGB, 2006). Routine screening is carried out at a GP surgery; however, the availability of more flexible appointment times in a community pharmacy setting means that patients can keep to appointment times more readily, which reduces the workload at the GP practice allowing nursing staff to treat more seriously ill patients.

The future of the community pharmacist

The development of additional professional roles has enhanced pharmacists' roles within the team of health professionals. 'Medicines management' involves a range of activities intended to improve the way that medicines are used, by patients and by the NHS (see Chapter 6 for more information). Medicines management services are processes based on patient need that are used to design, implement, deliver and monitor patient-focused care. 'Priorities for Action' developed in 2004 by the Department of Health, Social Services and Public Safety (DHSSPS) for the UK and Northern Ireland, made a priority of 'Working for Healthier People', giving a budget commitment to developing the role of the community pharmacist further, modernising and improving services, promoting integrated working across primary, secondary and community sectors and improving efficiency and performance. Priorities for Action has endorsed the development of a medicines management service in order to start making full use of community pharmacists' skills (DHSSPS, 2006). Areas where community pharmacy can contribute to the medicines management agenda include:

- ongoing medication review
- improving patient understanding and use of prescribed medication
- developing care programmes and services for 'at risk' patient groups
- protocols for patient counselling and self-medication
- health promotion and multidisciplinary research
- audit and drug utilisation review.

It is also important to note the substantial role pharmacists play in providing prescribing support. In this context, pharmacists work at different levels: individual practice, local health and social care group, and health and social services board. These pharmacists also contribute to the medicines management agenda. Examples of the key areas of involvement include:

- prescribing analysis and feedback
- formulary development and maintenance
- review and management of repeat prescribing processes
- medication review.

Work is also under way to develop prescribing policies across the primary–secondary care interface, and across the whole of the pharmaceutical sector, developing opportunities for pharmacist prescribing allied to the *Crown Report* (1999).

Pharmacy practice has been evolving to meet the needs of a contemporary healthcare system. The modern role of the community pharmacist is well articulated in the *Report of the Joint Working Party on the Future Role of the Community Pharmaceutical Service*, published in 1992 (Hawksworth & Chrystyn, 1992). In addition, a major and ongoing initiative by the RPSGB – 'Pharmacy in a New Age', started in 1995 – seeks to set out what pharmacy does and can offer, supported by information technology, education and training, audit and research.

References

British Society for the History of Pharmacy (2007). www.bshp.org (accessed 5 March 2007).

CIPPET – Centre for Inter-Professional Postgraduate Education and Training; www.pharmacy.rdg.ac.uk/cippet (accessed 5 March 2007).

CPPE – Centre for Pharmacy Postgraduate Education – www.cppe.manchester.ac.uk

Crown Report (1999). *Review of Prescribing, Supply and Administration of Medicines. Final report.* www.jcn.co.uk/pdf/crownreport2.pdf (accessed 5 March 2007).

Department of Health (2007). *Patient Group Directions* http://www.dh.gov.uk/en/Policyandguidance/Emergencyplanning/DH_4069610 (accessed 5 March 2007).

DHSSPS (2006). *Priorities for Action.* Department of Health and Social Services and the Pharmaceutical Service for Northern Ireland. www.dhsspsni.gov.uk/pfa_2007–08.pdf (accessed 5 March 2007).

Hawksworth GM, Chrystyn H. (1992). Clinical pharmacy in primary care. *Br J Clin Pharmacol* 46: 415–420.

IC (2006). *Prescriptions Dispensed, 2005*. http:// www.ic.nhs.uk/statistics-and-data-collections/ primary-care/prescribing/prescriptions-dispensed-2005. Information Centre for Health and Social Care (accessed 5 March 2007).

IC (2007). *National Prescribing Costs and Items*. www.ic.nhs.uk/statistics-and-data-collections/ primary-care/prescriptions (accessed 5 March 2007).

National Prescribing Centre (2007). *Clinical Governance*. www.npc.co.uk/publications/auditHandbook/ clinical_gov.htm (accessed 26 February 2007).

Taylor K M G, Harding G, eds (2001). *Pharmacy Practice*. Taylor & Francis.

Parliamentary Office of Science and Technology (2005). *Changing Role of Pharmacies*. www. parliament.uk/documents/upload/postpn246.pdf Parliamentary Office of Science and Technology (accessed 26 February 2007).

Royal Pharmaceutical Society of Great Britain (2006). *Diagnostic Testing in Community Pharmacy*. www. rpsgb.org.uk/pdfs/rpsepicdiagtest.pdf (accessed 5 March 2007).

United Nations (2001). *World Population Ageing: 1950– 2050* www.un.org/esa/population/publications/ worldageing19502050/pdf/preface_web.pdf (accessed 26 February 2007).

4

An overview of hospital pharmacy

Kate E Fletcher

Introduction

This chapter introduces hospital pharmacy and describes the roles of the pharmacist and other pharmacy staff within the hospital setting, clinical pharmacy (the role of the pharmacist and other pharmacy staff on hospital wards), the specialities that pharmacists can work in within hospital pharmacy and future developments for hospital pharmacy.

Traditional roles of the hospital pharmacist

Until about 30 years ago, pharmacists in UK hospitals were to be found in the dispensary, processing stock orders and prescriptions, and rarely setting foot outside of the pharmacy department, except to perform 'ward pharmacy', which at this stage was little more than collecting dispensing work from wards. Consequently, the traditional roles of the hospital pharmacist were dispensing and supplying stock drugs to wards and departments. Many products were made extemporaneously (Box 4.1), and therefore most departments had an in-house quality control (QC) section. QC, or quality assurance (QA) as it is now more often called, involves testing pharmaceutical products to ensure they are safe and suitable for use. These tests may therefore investigate aspects such as sterility or composition. QA also ensures that unlicensed medicines (Box 4.1) ordered by the pharmacy department are manufactured to the appropriate standards before being supplied for use in patients (see below).

In the early 1970s, with the development of clinical pharmacy and the increasing role of the pharmacy technician, pharmacists started moving out of the dispensary to work side by side with nurses and doctors on wards. As a result, the role of the hospital pharmacist in the 21st century would be barely recognisable to the pharmacist of 50 years ago because rather than the pharmacist being confined to the pharmacy

---

Box 4.1   Definitions of terms used in Chapter 4

Accredited checking technician

Technicians may be accredited by a nationally recognised training scheme to carry out the final accuracy check of dispensed items clinically approved by a registered pharmacist.

Extemporaneous product

In the context of medicinal products, an extemporaneous product or preparation is not pre-prepared; it is made on site, at the time of need, for an individual patient, based on a prescription (see Chapter 14).

Final accuracy check of a dispensed prescription

This process ensures that the item selected and labelled matches the prescription in every detail: drug, strength, dose, frequency and name of patient; this check may be carried out by a registered pharmacist, or an accredited checking technician.

Therapeutics

This is the branch of medicine concerned with the treatment of disease, using medicines rather than surgery.

Unlicensed medicine

An unlicensed medicine does not have a marketing authorisation (MA). In the UK, all medicines go through strict checks to make sure that they are safe and effective. When the medicine passes all the required checks, an MA (formerly known as a product licence) is granted, which means that the medicine can be used in the treatment of specific medical conditions. Pharmaceutical manufacturers must apply to the Medicines and Healthcare products Regulatory Agency (MHRA) for an MA if they want to sell their medicines in the UK. The MHRA approves the product licence for a medicine if it has been proven to work for the illnesses it was developed for, does not have too many side-effects or risks and has been made to a high standard.

---

department, they are now to be found in all parts of the hospital; on ward rounds with doctors, in the Accident and Emergency Department, in operating theatres and outpatient clinics.

The structure of a typical hospital pharmacy department

There are many roles within a hospital pharmacy department, only some of which are performed by pharmacists. While pharmacists are responsible for all professional aspects of the work of a pharmacy (i.e. ensuring the output of the department is safe and legal), technicians are responsible for a large proportion of that output: dispensing prescriptions, managing pharmacy stores and preparing sterile products. The role of technicians has also developed in recent years to include medicines management (see Chapter 6), medicines information (MI; see page 39), information technology support (maintaining pharmacy computer systems) and final checking of

prescriptions (accredited checking technicians) (Box 4.1). Some technicians are also moving into roles such as dispensary management (see page 38). Thus, the roles of the hospital pharmacist and hospital pharmacy technician are becoming increasingly interdependent.

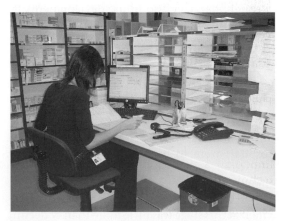

Figure 4.1   A clinical pharmacist screens a prescription chart.

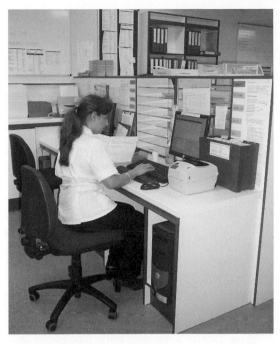

Figure 4.2   A pharmacy technician produces labels for a prescription.

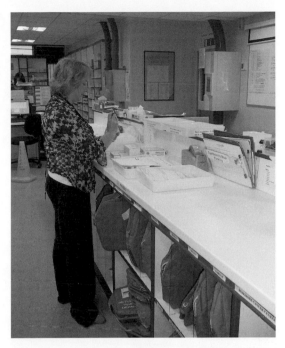

Figure 4.4   A pharmacist performs the final technical check of a discharge prescription.

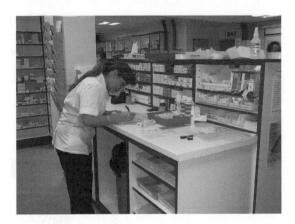

Figure 4.3   A pharmacy technician dispenses a discharge prescription.

Assistant technical officers (ATOs) play an important supportive role to pharmacists and technicians. They may be dispensary receptionists, for example, receiving work into the dispensary and answering the telephone; some ATOs are trained to dispense prescriptions and prepare sterile products; others may work in pharmacy stores, preparing stock orders for wards and departments. All wards and clinical departments within a hospital (i.e. areas that treat patients) have a stock of the drugs and equipment that are used regularly in that area. The stock drugs are listed on a pharmacy stock list, and staff in that area can order any item on the stock list from the pharmacy; these orders are processed in the pharmacy stores, and then delivered to the department that made the order.

Pharmacists, technicians and ATOs work side by side in the pharmacy, and tend to have parallel management structures. Pharmacists are usually managed by a more senior pharmacist, and technicians and ATOs are usually managed by a more senior technician. Most departments have a senior management team which is composed of the chief pharmacist, deputy chief pharmacist, clinical services manager and operational manager, and which oversees all parts of the department. The role of the chief pharmacist is described below. The deputy chief pharmacist may also be the clinical services manager or operational manager, or share some of the roles and responsibilities of the chief pharmacist. The

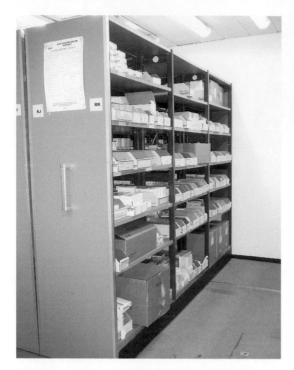

Figure 4.5   Shelving in a typical hospital pharmacy stores.

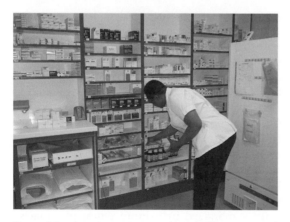

Figure 4.6   A senior assistant technical officer puts stock away in the dispensary.

clinical services manager is a senior pharmacist responsible for the services provided by the pharmacy to wards and other clinical areas, and will usually manage all the other pharmacists. The operational manager is either a senior pharmacist or technician, and is responsible for the

efficient operation of the pharmacy department. The operational manager will usually manage the technicians and ATOs.

Clinical pharmacy

Clinical pharmacy, that is, the practice of pharmacy 'at the bedside', or at least, on wards and in clinical departments, started to develop in the USA in the late 1960s and in the UK during the 1970s. Initially, pharmacists performing ward pharmacy did little more than collect stock orders and transcribe patient-specific drug orders from drug charts, engaging in little contact with doctors, nurses or patients. Gradually, pharmacists started to use their expert pharmaceutical knowledge to monitor prescribing, intervening when appropriate to optimise drug treatment for individual patients. Now, many hospital pharmacists are fully integrated into the clinical team, working alongside doctors, nurses, physiotherapists and other members of the multidisciplinary team, to deliver optimal care to patients. With the pharmacist present at the time of prescribing, errors in selection of appropriate drug and dosing regimen are minimised, ensuring that the patient receives maximum benefit from their treatment with minimal side-effects.

Pharmaceutical care

Pharmaceutical care is the term most often used to describe what a clinical pharmacist does. It entails regular monitoring of drug treatment for each patient under their care, including screening prescription charts for safety, appropriateness, efficacy and side-effects.

Concepts and definitions in clinical pharmacy are changing frequently. Over the years, different jargon has been used to describe the work of the clinical pharmacist. In 1990, Hepler and Strand defined the concept of pharmaceutical care for the first time as 'the responsible provision of drug therapy for the purpose of achieving definite outcomes that improve a patient's quality of life'.

The process of pharmaceutical care can be carried out in a variety of ways. Most clinical pharmacists have responsibility for particular wards; they will make regular visits (usually daily, Monday to Friday) to these wards to carry out a pharmacist ward round, which involves inspecting each patient's prescription chart, as described above, and, when necessary, observation charts and medical notes. During these rounds, the pharmacist will talk with the patient to confirm details such as medication history, when and how a patient takes their medication, and also to enquire whether certain medication, such as antiemetics (drugs to prevent and treat nausea and vomiting) or analgesics (painkillers) are working and being tolerated. In order to perform effectively, the pharmacist must have good communication skills to gather all the information they need from both patients and other health professionals (see Chapter 8).

Most pharmacy departments have an out-of-hours on-call system. These systems vary from a residency service, where a small team of resident pharmacists (often junior grades) take turns (on a rota) to stay on site over night in order to provide a complete pharmaceutical supply and advice service, to an 'at home' on-call service, where all the pharmacists in a department take turns (on a rota) to provide an 'emergency only' service. In this system, pharmacists go home at the end of the working day, but hospital staff can contact the pharmacist for advice via a pager. There is usually an 'emergency drug cupboard' at the hospital that contains drugs that are not available elsewhere in the hospital and that nurses and doctors can access out of hours. A residency service offers a similar level of service to that available during the working day; an 'emergency only' service offers help and supply of drugs only when it is vital that there is no delay in treatment. The on-call service offered by a pharmacy department is usually determined by the amount of funding available for the service; clearly it is more expensive to run a residency service, as more pharmacists are needed to support it, and not all trusts have sufficient funds to support this.

Many clinical pharmacists participate in doctors' ward rounds. This enables the pharmacist to obtain greater in-depth knowledge of a patient's condition, and to have a direct influence on prescribing – being present when a therapeutic decision is made enables the pharmacist to ensure that the choice of drug is appropriate for the patient *before* the prescription is written. The pharmacist can also ensure the drug is available, so the patient's treatment is not delayed. This combination of prescribing advice and supply of medication ensures timely and safe treatment and improves patient care.

Pharmacists also help and advise nurses on the safe administration and monitoring of drug treatment, discuss possible food–drug interactions with dietitians, and ascertain from speech and language therapists whether a patient can swallow medications safely.

Pharmacists may also participate in outpatient clinics. Pharmacists are frequently involved in anticoagulant clinics, where they are responsible for checking patients' blood results, advising on warfarin dose adjustment, and counselling new patients on their warfarin treatment. (Warfarin is an anticoagulant drug – it reduces the ability of the blood to form clots. Warfarin is used in conditions that increase the risk of the blood clotting such as atrial fibrillation.)

Teaching

Hospital pharmacists begin teaching one another as soon as they enter their pre-registration training – through case and project presentations they teach their peers and other members of the pharmacy department about specific drugs, conditions, or project design and execution, such as audit technique. Carrying out these presentations is a requirement of the pre-registration training programme; they are also essential skills for the hospital pharmacist, and are an integral part of improving the communication skills essential for a pharmacist's everyday work.

As hospital pharmacists become more experienced and specialised (see below), part of their responsibility is likely to be the teaching and training of other pharmacists, nurses and doctors. Senior pharmacists tutor junior pharmacists studying for postgraduate qualifications such as a diploma in clinical pharmacy – the senior pharmacist acts as mentor and tutor, helping the 'diploma pharmacist' achieve their goals. Diplomas in clinical pharmacy are offered by several universities in the UK, including – but not limited to – Cardiff University, University of Derby, Keele University, the University of London and Queen's University Belfast. There are also opportunities for hospital pharmacists to specialise in departmental or regional teaching and training, by presenting to local area (branch) (see Chapter 7) meetings, or at local specialist training days.

Most schools of pharmacy in the UK employ teacher practitioners (TPs) – practising pharmacists who are also members of academic staff. They may come from any sector of pharmacy (i.e. community, hospital, primary care, industry) and contribute up-to-date knowledge and experience of practice to the course content, giving undergraduates an invaluable insight to current practice. TPs may also advise full-time academic staff on various aspects of teaching and course content, to ensure it is relevant to practice, and act as a liaison between academia and their own particular sector of practice, to facilitate undergraduate visits and training placements. For instance, a visit to a pharmaceutical company manufacturing plant might be arranged, or students might undertake a placement in a community pharmacy or hospital pharmacy department, to gain experience and knowledge of working in those environments. TPs also establish links between institutions for research and educational purposes.

Specialisation in hospital pharmacy

Clinical specialisation

Pharmacists can specialise in many clinical areas. Most large National Health Service trusts will have specialist pharmacist posts in areas such as cardiology, critical care, elderly care, gastroenterology, general medicine, haematology, oncology, paediatrics, renal medicine, surgery, trauma and orthopaedics.

As well as being experts in the therapeutics (Box 4.1) relating to their speciality, these pharmacists are often responsible for producing reports that analyse prescribing patterns and spending on medicines and developing prescribing guidelines in partnership with clinicians. They may also manage junior pharmacists or pharmacy technicians working within their speciality.

Pharmacy specialisation

Some pharmacists choose a non-clinical speciality. These include dispensary manager, education and training, MI, QA, and sterile and non-sterile production.

Dispensary management

The dispensary is the heart of the hospital pharmacy, and as such needs to be run efficiently to ensure that the right drug gets to the right patient at the right time. Dispensaries have traditionally been managed by pharmacists, but with the development of the role of the pharmacy technician in recent years, many dispensaries are now 'technician led'. Accredited checking technicians (see Box 4.1) are able to take on more of the pharmacist's role, performing the technical check of a dispensed prescription. This has reduced the number of pharmacists needed to run a dispensary, allowing them to devote more time to clinical activity, and therefore makes better use of their training and expertise.

Education and training

All staff within a pharmacy department, especially pharmacists and technicians, must keep up-to-date with recent developments in their profession. Indeed, during the next few years continuing professional development (CPD) will become mandatory for pharmacists and technicians to retain their registration.

To facilitate CPD, many pharmacy departments have designated pharmacists and technicians who are responsible for assessing the education and training needs of the staff. They are often also responsible for managing the training and assessment programmes for pre-registration pharmacists and student technicians.

When newly registered pharmacists (junior pharmacists) start work in a hospital pharmacy, they will often enter a clinical training rotation. This involves working in different areas within the pharmacy department (such as MI (see below), dispensary, or sterile production) and on different wards, for periods (or rotations) of 3–4 months; this enables the junior pharmacist to gain experience and skills in different areas of pharmacy and different clinical specialities.

To progress in a career as a hospital pharmacist, it is now more or less mandatory to have a postgraduate qualification in clinical pharmacy. This is usually undertaken by junior pharmacists when they start on a clinical training rotation, and takes 2–3 years part time. Several universities offer such courses (see above), and individual pharmacy departments tend to send all their junior pharmacists on the same course, so that it is easier to provide support to the students and to plan work rotas when the group is away on study days, etc., at the same time. The course content is delivered in a variety of ways, such as fortnightly regional study days, weekly 2 hour training sessions or week-long residential courses. This is supplemented by course work, which usually includes case studies and presentations, patient profiles and audit projects. Most courses also include exams.

Most pharmacists will study to diploma level; however, it is becoming more common for pharmacists to obtain a masters degree in clinical pharmacy. These are offered alongside the postgraduate diploma.

As well as formal courses, hospital pharmacy departments take advantage of study days provided both within their trust and by other trusts. These might involve learning generic skills such as time management, dealing with difficult situations and people management, or might be run by pharmacy staff for pharmacy staff, covering subjects and skills unique to pharmacy, such as clinical pharmacy skills or medicines management topics.

Another way pharmacists and technicians can maintain their knowledge is to attend symposia and conferences relevant to their area of practice. Many such conferences take place around the world each year, providing a useful forum for pharmacy staff to hear up-to-the-minute presentations from international experts, and to meet other practitioners and exchange ideas and information. Within the UK, popular conferences for clinical pharmacists are the British Pharmaceutical Conference (BPC), run by the Royal Pharmaceutical Society of Great Britain (RPSGB), and conferences and symposia run by the UK Clinical Pharmacy Association (UKCPA) and the Guild of Healthcare Pharmacists (GHP). Specialist conferences include the annual symposium of the British Oncology Pharmacy Association (BOPA).

Medicines information

MI is a service provided by pharmacists and technicians in many pharmacy departments for other pharmacists, other health professionals such as doctors and nurses, and, in some departments, members of the public.

The MI service has developed alongside clinical pharmacy to support clinical pharmacists. MI provides in-depth information on all aspects of drug use. The staff within MI use medical and pharmaceutical texts (e.g. *Martindale: The Complete Drug Reference*, Trissel's *Handbook on Injectable Drugs*, Stockley's *Drug Interactions*), pharmaceutical companies and online databases (such as PubMed and Pharmline) to research queries made by the service users. Examples of enquiries include:

- Is drug X safe for use during pregnancy?
- Does drug Y interact with drug Z?
- Can drug A be given intravenously, and if so, how should it be given?

Details of these reference books and online databases are provided on page 41.

Quality assurance

Pharmaceutical products must be of high quality to ensure patient safety and efficacy of treatment. The production of pharmaceutical products in the UK is governed by the *Rules and Guidance for Pharmaceutical Manufacturers and Distributors* published by the Medicines and Healthcare products Regulatory Agency (MHRA) (also known as the 'Orange Guide' because of the orange cover). All pharmaceutical products licensed for use in the UK are manufactured and tested according to the *Orange Guide* by the manufacturers, and therefore can be assumed to be of suitable quality when received by a pharmacy. Unlicensed products may not be subject to the *Orange Guide* however, and there must therefore be a mechanism in place to ascertain the quality of these products. For hospital pharmacies, this is carried out by a QA department. Hospitals can have their own QA department, but in some regions QA services have been centralised to reduce costs, one department serving several hospitals. The staff within this department are often pharmacists and pharmacy technicians, but may also be other scientists and laboratory technicians. All must have the appropriate skills and knowledge to carry out quantitative and qualitative testing on a range of pharmaceutical products, including medicines in various formulations, and medical gases. QA staff are also involved in risk management and clinical governance.

Sterile and non-sterile production

Historically, many hospital pharmacy departments had a production unit that made many different sterile (such as bladder irrigation fluids and eye drops) and non-sterile (such as creams, ointments and liquid medicines) pharmaceutical

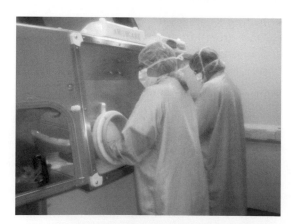

Figure 4.7 Pharmacy technicians producing sterile dispensed items in an aseptic unit.

products. With the emergence of a far greater range of commercially manufactured products available since the 1980s, many of these units have greatly reduced output or have been closed down.

Some production units do remain in hospitals, however, and most commonly they will prepare products with a short shelf life, on an individual patient basis, for instance chemotherapy used in the treatment of cancer.

Such units are staffed by pharmacists, pharmacy technicians and ATOs who have specialised in this area of practice. It is increasingly common for technicians to manage these units, rather than pharmacists. Junior staff from the pharmacy department often work in the production unit for a few months as part of a training rotation, to gain some knowledge and skills in this area.

Management

Each area within the hospital pharmacy requires a manager. As discussed above, this may be a pharmacist or technician, depending on the skills that are required for the post. Management roles often filled by technicians include dispensary manager and sterile production manager. Roles such as clinical services manager and medicines information manager are usually filled by pharmacists.

The department as a whole is usually led by a chief pharmacist, who will typically have worked in various areas within hospital pharmacy and so have a broad understanding of how it works. They also need to have good communication and time- and people-management skills. They are likely to have been registered for a minimum of 10 years. The chief pharmacist takes overall responsibility for the work of all the staff within the department; he or she is responsible for ensuring that the work carried out by the department meets the legal and ethical standards laid out in the legislature (e.g. the Medicines Act 1968), and in *Medicines, Ethics and Practice Guide for Pharmacists and Pharmacy Technicians*. The Chief Pharmacist is also answerable to the trust's management with regard to the services provided by the pharmacy department.

The future of hospital pharmacy

With the introduction of supplementary and independent prescribing, pharmacists have the opportunity to enhance their existing skills and to expand the ways in which they use them, to the benefit of patients. As pharmacists move into these extended roles, pharmacy technicians and ATOs are developing their skills and knowledge to take on roles previously fulfilled by pharmacists.

The future of hospital pharmacy will see the continuation of the development of patient-centred care. The introduction of new technologies, such as electronic prescribing and robotic dispensing, will enable pharmacy staff to spend more time on patient-focused activities to improve the outcome of treatment.

Summary

Hospital pharmacy offers a wide-ranging and challenging career for the newly qualified pharmacist, using many of the skills and much of the knowledge acquired at university.

This chapter provides the student with an understanding of what this career offers and the roles available in the hospital pharmacy: practising in a multidisciplinary team as a specialist clinical pharmacist, managing a sterile production unit, running the MI centre, or moving into a management role, such as dispensary manager, clinical services manager or even becoming a chief pharmacist. Underpinning all of these roles is the fundamental role of the pharmacist, which is to ensure that the patient receives the best pharmaceutical care possible, maximising benefit from the medicines they receive.

References

Hepler C D, Strand L M (1990). Opportunities and responsibilities in pharmaceutical care. *Am J Hosp Pharm* 47: 533–543.

Useful resources

Baxter K, ed (2007). *Stockley's Drug Interactions*, 8th edn. London: Pharmaceutical Press.

Medicines and Healthcare products Regulatory Agency (2007). *Rules and Guidance for Pharmaceutical Manufacturers and Distributors*. London: Pharmaceutical Press (the so-called *Orange Guide*).

Pharmline (Database for medicines management, prescribing and pharmacy): www.pharm-line.nhs.uk

PubMed (reference database provided by the US National Library of Medicine): http://www.ncbi.nlm.nih.gov/sites/entrez?db=PubMed

Royal Pharmaceutical Society of Great Britain (2007). *Medicines, Ethics and Practice: A Guide For Pharmacists and Pharmacy Technicians*, 31st edn. London: Pharmaceutical Press.

Sweetman S C, ed (2006). *Martindale: The Complete Drug Reference,* 35th edn. London: Pharmaceutical Press.

Trissel L A (2007). *Handbook on Injectable Drugs*, 14th edn. Transatlantic Publishing.

5

An overview of industrial sector pharmacy

Clare F Rawlinson

Introduction

The role of the pharmacist as a distinct entity separate from the physician has emerged over the course of history. At its inception, this role involved the compounding of medicinal products, including chemist's nostrums and extemporaneously prepared items (see Chapter 14). Over time, this local preparation of medicines within individual pharmacies, whether to a formula prescribed by the doctor or by the pharmacist, has diminished. These formulations have been replaced by products developed, licensed and manufactured by companies with specific expertise in these areas. The majority of medicinal products dispensed to patients nowadays are prepared by central manufacturing processes performed by pharmaceutical companies.

This centralised development 'pipeline' for medicinal products has allowed a large range of new chemical entities (NCEs) to be discovered and more complicated dosage forms and devices to be developed. Potential NCEs must pass through a complex series of regulated clinical trials in order to become licensed and proceed to market. This strict framework aims to assess the safety and efficacy of these products and to prevent severe or unacceptable side-effects for potential patients. Pharmaceutical companies have various departments, employing people with particular skill sets, which deal with these different stages of getting a new drug successfully to the market. This development pipeline provides the benefit of effective, quality-assured and 'safe' medicines to the population. (Note: safety is subjective – no drug is truly safe. All drugs show some adverse effects or side-effects in some patient populations.) The drug development process aims to address previously untreatable conditions and improve on the treatments currently provided for other disease states.

Within their undergraduate training, pharmacists study a wide range of subjects. These include:

- medicinal chemistry – the design, synthesis and development of pharmaceutical drugs

- pharmacology – how substances interact with living organisms to change their function
- pharmaceutics – the science of dosage form design, i.e. the processes of turning an NCE (drug) into a safe and efficacious medicine.

This gives qualified pharmacists a unique breadth of knowledge and skill profile that is particularly useful within the pharmaceutical industry. The pharmacist is therefore well qualified to play a key role within a network of multidisciplinary professionals at each stage of the drug development process (Wicks, 2000). This chapter describes some of the major areas where these opportunities arise.

Research and development

Research and development (R&D) covers the whole process of making a drug compound into a viable dosage form to be taken by or administered to a patient. At the beginning of this process of discovery, the basic structure of a lead (or parent) compound that has promising therapeutic effects can be modified by using different methods of synthesis. These changes (e.g. to chemical side group) can make the drug target a specific receptor or site more accurately. Many NCEs with slight modifications in structure are synthesised. These are then rapidly analysed for therapeutic potential and favourable physical properties using specialised high-throughput screening techniques. This process is managed by a scientist with a speciality in medicinal chemistry.

Once a promising NCE is identified, it will be passed to the formulation department. This is the stage of R&D where the majority of pharmacists are employed. The NCE is transformed from a pure, usually powdered, drug compound to a formulation that can be administered to a patient, for example by intravenous injection or as a tablet. The preferred route of administration is usually oral (i.e. tablet or capsule). This route does not involve the risk of infection associated with subcutaneous or intravenous injection and is easy for the patient to administer themselves. However, an intravenous formulation will often

be developed first for early clinical trials (see page 47).

In order to obtain a therapeutic response to a drug, an adequate concentration of the drug needs to be delivered to and maintained at the site(s) of action (Proudfoot, 1988). The amount of drug at the site of action relative to the dose administered is termed the bioavailability. This is affected by many factors once the drug is in the body (e.g. degradation, elimination and absorption) which in turn are influenced by the physicochemical characteristics of the compound. These characteristics may hinder delivery by a particular route (e.g. a product that doesn't dissolve in aqueous solutions is difficult to deliver in an oral formulation). The formulation scientist may modify the NCE to improve these physicochemical characteristics, which may be through selection of a different drug salt or a polymorphic form with different solubility, physical state or stability. Alternatively, they may add carefully selected excipients that improve the delivery of the drug compound (e.g. by improving its dissolution profile).

This area of development may involve many dosage forms: tablets, capsules, solutions and suspensions for oral administration; creams, ointments and transdermal patches; inhalers; suppositories and enemas; injectable solutions; eye and ear drops. During development of these products a formulation will be established and a manufacturing technique developed. The scientists involved will be interested in achieving effective delivery and good bioavailability from products, as well as ensuring adequate stability for the lifetime of the product.

Formulation scientists also work on established drug compounds to improve or modify their delivery. Examples include modified-release preparations such as sustained-release painkillers or antidiabetic drugs that allow less frequent dosing of the medicine. This can produce a more convenient product, improving patient adherence and therefore efficacy of the treatment. Delivery of established drug compounds through novel routes of administration, with associated benefits of this new route, is another area of development. A recent example of this is the delivery of insulin via an inhaler device. This avoids the pain of injection, the traditional route of administration. These new products also result in new patents for the pharmaceutical company, with associated revenue.

A sub-speciality within this field of formulation has emerged with the development of biotechnology. This involves the delivery of vaccines, proteins, DNA and drug molecules to the body through a variety of 'smart' devices or targeted delivery. This includes products often described under the umbrella of 'nanotechnology'.

The pharmacist has a unique integrated understanding of physiology, pharmacology and chemistry, making them ideally placed to understand the relationship between drug structure, formulation and bioavailability and, in addition, to integrate concepts of patient acceptability into this development process. They therefore work successfully alongside chemists and pharmacologists, throughout the R&D process.

A relevant PhD is desirable for a career in this area of industrial pharmacy. Depending on the subject studied, this develops a knowledge base specific to medicinal chemistry and/or formulation and, in addition, project management and strategic problem-solving skills. Pharmaceutical companies will often support employees to pursue a part-time postgraduate degree by research alongside employment.

Manufacturing

Small-scale manufacturing is performed during formulation development within the R&D department. However, when a product moves on to full-scale manufacture problems may arise

---

Box 5.1   Case study: Research and development formulation

I studied Pharmacy at Trinity College Dublin, graduating in 1993. After registering, I was keen to start working so I got a job in community pharmacy. Then (as now), this branch of pharmacy had the highest starting salaries. After 3 years, 2 of which involved managing a pharmacy, I decided that I needed more of a challenge.

I was fortunate to get my start in industry as a formulation scientist in their new technologies department at Elan Pharmaceutical Technologies. Elan specialised in delivering 'old' drugs in new ways (e.g. formulating a three-times-a-day drug as once daily) and in developing new routes of delivery (e.g. trying to make oral formulations of injectable drugs). From this job I gained extensive practical experience both in a laboratory setting and in good manufacturing practice, and a valuable introduction to how challenging busy projects can be.

After 2 years with Elan, I decided that gaining a PhD would be a logical step if I wished to progress my career in research and development. I was fortunate to be offered an industry-sponsored PhD with the University of Nottingham, looking at the use of a novel absorption enhancer, chitosan, for the oral delivery of poorly bioavailable drugs such as insulin. Studying for the PhD gave me an excellent hands-on way of building my scientific confidence and improving my problem-solving skills. After getting my PhD, I worked for a start-up drug delivery company investigating novel gastroretentive technologies.

In 2005, I began my current job as a senior scientist in the formulation department at Bristol-Myers Squibb. I work with people of different disciplines in different geographical locations, and the work ranges from practical work to report writing to formal presentations, with ample opportunity for travel. The company places a strong emphasis on career development.

For me personally, I have found pharmacist roles in industry to offer far greater challenges and variety than working in community pharmacy, and opportunities for career progression offer a huge choice. My advice for a young graduate starting out would be to try out different jobs, and to look beyond tempting starting salaries to find something you really enjoy doing.

Dr Michael Leane

Senior Scientist, Pharmaceutics Research and Development, Bristol-Myers Squibb

at any stage of production; poor flow of powders from hoppers, segregation of mixed powders during movement of materials between stages of manufacture, and incorrect granulation mixture consistency are just some examples of the problems that may be encountered during tabletting.

Pharmacists are often involved in the product transfer process (i.e. from the formulation laboratory to the manufacturing plant). They can apply knowledge of pharmaceutics to deduce the cause of a problem. This information can be used to make slight alterations to the formulation whilst liaising with the R&D department to solve the particular problem without adversely affecting the final performance of the product.

Quality assurance

Quality assurance is an important part of the manufacturing process, and pharmacists often become involved in this area. Quality is a concept that means different things to different people. In relation to pharmaceutical products it means that the product is fit for purpose – it is fit to be given to a patient in the confidence that it will have the desired effects and will not harm or damage him of her in any way, through faults of manufacture (Sharp, 1994). Quality assurance involves testing the raw material and manufactured product at different stages to ensure

---

Box 5.2   Case study: Manufacturing

I studied Pharmacy at John Moore's University Liverpool and graduated in July 2004. I enjoyed all aspects of the degree course but particularly the Industrial Pharmacy module and my final year project, which was a study of dosage form design, in which I looked at the tabletting properties of various grades of hydroxypropylmethylcellulose (HPMC) and lactose.

I completed my pre-registration year in the community sector and, following registration, I spent a further 6 months as a relief manager, and then a permanent manager, for the same firm. Whilst enjoying my time in community pharmacy, I realised that I wanted to use more of the knowledge gained at university, so I decided to move into the industrial sector. I became a scientist in the pharmaceutical development group at Bristol-Myers Squibb (BMS).

Since beginning at BMS I have been involved in a number of different projects, each at a different stage in the drug development programme. Working on various projects has provided variety, as well as very

useful experience. No two days are ever exactly alike. Typical activities range from small- to medium-scale manufacturing (using a wide range of equipment), dissolution testing and recording, reporting and summarising the resultant data.

Non-project related activities include the calibration and validation of equipment, audit, setting up and chairing a Pharmacist forum within the company, and being a representative on a number of sub-teams related to electronic laboratory notebooks.

Working in industry has allowed me to use much of the knowledge gained on my degree course, whilst presenting a constant and interesting challenge. BMS places strong emphasis on high-quality training, team work and cooperation whilst enabling individuals to plan and take responsibility for their own work.

Michael Thompson

Scientist, Pharmaceutics Research and Development, Bristol-Myers Squibb

that the desired quality is achieved. Examples include testing the mix quality of a physical mix or granulation, the strength of a granule or the friability of a final tablet product.

As part of this assurance process, good manufacturing practice (GMP) guidelines must be adhered to. These involve a strict method of working, with standard operating procedures (SOPs) for manufacture and clean down, accompanied by supporting documentation at each stage of the process. Within these guidelines a medicinal product is fit for purpose when it:

- is the right product
- is the right strength
- is free from contamination
- has in no way deteriorated or broken down
- is in the right container
- is correctly labelled
- is properly sealed in its container and protected against damage and contamination.

The aim of these processes is to build 'quality by design' into the manufacturing processes. It is not possible to test each item manufactured, but there are dangers to patients even if only a small number of defective items are released for consumption. Put simply, this means that products (and processes) are designed to be 'good' and to meet specifications, rather than testing at the point of manufacture to ensure that it is not 'bad' or out of specifications.

Stability testing of the product also falls within the remit of this discipline. This involves testing drug formulations under accelerated conditions (i.e. at higher than ambient temperatures and pressures). Extrapolation of this data to room temperature allows the prediction of how long the product will remain stable (and viable for administration to a patient). The expiry date of a marketed product is then decided on the basis of this data.

Many pharmacists working in this sector are now choosing to take the 'qualified person' (QP) qualification. The primary role of the QP is to ensure that each batch of a medicinal product has been manufactured or assembled and checked in compliance with the provisions of the

law. The QP authorises the release of each manufactured batch, and is also involved in ensuring the standards and completion of appropriate paperwork for imported and exported raw materials and final drug formulations. This professional qualification involves specific postgraduate training; it is much sought after by pharmaceutical companies, as it is a legal requirement for the manufacture and supply of drugs for clinical trials (Wicks, 2000).

Clinical trials

Clinical trials are a controlled investigation of a clinical treatment. This may include pharmaceutical medications, vaccines, medical devices, surgical techniques, clinical practice or 'nutraceuticals'. Here we will focus on the testing of pharmaceuticals. Within a clinical trial, drugs are tested in human volunteers to establish optimal dosing, efficacy and safety. Before this, any NCE will have undergone preclinical testing: cell culture tests, animal studies, toxicology, potential effectiveness, gross (severe) side-effects, and pharmacological and toxicity testing in animal subjects. These results are reviewed by regulatory authorities. Many compounds are rejected at this stage (by either the pharmaceutical company or a regulatory authority) because of an unfavourable toxicity profile; only the most promising compounds are tested in humans.

Before starting a trial, approval must be sought from the Medicines and Healthcare products Regulatory Agency (MHRA) in the UK or other relevant licensing authority (see section on Regulatory affairs, page 50). Approval is also required from the National Research Ethics (NRE) service. Trials are reviewed by an appointed NRE committee, at least one member of which must be a pharmacist. Issues discussed may include whether the benefit of the treatment outweighs the risk to the patient, which will vary depending on the disease state, patient age and whether treatment is for a chronic condition (e.g. asthma), or is likely to be short term (e.g. chemotherapy for life-threatening cancer). Other issues include the use of placebo as a comparator for serious or potentially serious diseases. In these cases it may be considered unethical to give patients a placebo (which is essentially withholding treatment) and the new treatment will be compared with the best alternative available on the market. The pharmacist uses his or her clinical, ethical and social knowledge to inform these decisions.

In Phase I trials, a single dose of the test drug is administered to a small number of healthy male volunteers, usually aged 18–60 years. The drug is often in an intravenous formulation at this stage in order to provide high bioavailability and so make efficacy evaluation more straightforward. Criteria assessed may include:

- tolerability – highest tolerated dose
- lowest effective dose
- dose–effect relationship
- duration of effect
- side-effects
- pharmacokinetics – time course of absorption, distribution and elimination).

A pharmacological effect is not necessarily observed however, depending on the drug under investigation, e.g. the effect of an antibiotic will not be seen in healthy volunteers.

Phase II trials are only performed if Phase I showed promising results. In a Phase II trial, the drug is tested in 100–300 volunteer patients with a specific indication. This is often performed in the patients' normal clinical environment (e.g. hospital or GP surgery). A therapeutic effect is expected in these patients and the following criteria are assessed:

- bioavailability
- efficacy
- side-effects
- pharmacokinetic data, which may differ from values in healthy volunteers because of the effect of the disease state
- interactions with current medication
- inter-patient variability (between different patients)
- intra-patient variability (in same patient at different times, e.g. affect of fasted state)
- risk–benefit ratio.

If adequate efficacy and advantages over standard therapy are shown in Phase II trials, and any risks from the treatment are acceptable, Phase III trials are performed. The drug is usually in its final or near-final formulation at this stage. The effects of the drug are evaluated in 1000–3000 volunteer patients who will be assessed and further information on safety and efficacy will be collected. The following will be established/assessed:

- set dosage
- type of administration
- some contraindications
- precautionary measures
- safety and efficacy on long-term use
- therapeutic advantage over established treatment
- clarification of interactions with other drugs.

If Phase III trials are successful, an application for marketing authorsation will be submitted.

Phase IV clinical trials (also called post-marketing surveillance) continue once the drug has received marketing authorisation and is available on prescription. These trials allow assessment of clinical data for:

- dosage optimisation
- drug–drug interactions
- identification of additional indications
- adverse effects associated with long-term use
- potential for overdose/misuse
- detailed evaluation of why some patients do not respond to the treatment
- long-term comparative data.

New dosage forms that allow patent extension may also be evaluated at this stage, including combination products of more than one NCE/drug.

Pharmacists are involved in all stages of clinical trials, starting with designing trial protocols and organising clinical trials supplies. They are involved in screening patients for suitability for inclusion in trials; they are ideally placed to assess criteria such a current drug usage and potential for drug interactions with concomitant medication. Pharmacists have good communication skills (see Chapter 9), which are vital in ensuring that patients give informed consent – each potential subject (patient) must be adequately informed of the aims, methods, anticipated benefits and potential hazards of the study, and the discomfort it may entail. Problems may occur in ensuring that subjects (patients/volunteers under study) understand, especially if the subject is a child or is incapacitated. Pharmacists may be employed by a pharmaceutical company or by the clinic running the trial (e.g. within a hospital setting).

Pharmacists may also participate in recruitment of patients (in contrast to the recruitment of healthy volunteers) whilst dealing with their routine treatment in the clinic. Pharmacists from all sectors of pharmacy also have a role to play in the Phase IV evaluation of medicines. They are an important partner in the reporting of suspected adverse reactions (side-effects) or unexpected events to the MHRA or other relevant body. In the UK, this is through the Yellow Card Scheme (see Chapter 4).

Medicines information

Medicines information (MI) is an important area of industrial pharmacy. Most pharmaceutical companies will have an MI department that holds information pertaining to their marketed drugs and sometimes for competitors' drugs as well. This is where data from all clinical trials and clinical reporting is collated and disseminated back to health professionals and the public. The MI department may also be asked to write technical literature for use by the company and to be involved in training medical representatives. The legal department within the company may also be involved in preparing and regulating the content of this information.

The MI department may act as a point of contact (further to the MHRA) for the reporting of adverse drug reactions by clinicians. This information is collated on to easily accessible databases and supplemented with online access to medical and scientific literature. The MI department will also field enquiries by doctors, pharmacists, nurses and patients. The information provided may include:

- alternative administration of the medicine, e.g. can a tablet be crushed for administration down a feeding tube without losing its efficacy? Can the drug be placed in a parenteral feed without binding to the ingredients and losing efficacy? Does this take its use outside of the product licence? (see Chapter 16)
- technical information about how to administer/use a medical device
- further details about contraindications, cautions and adverse drug reactions
- dosing in children or the elderly if this information is not currently available
- risk–benefit ratio of a particular drug treatment/adverse effect
- information about manufacturing and supply problems.

A pharmacist is ideally placed to perform these roles: they have clinical skills to understand the data available, and the communication skills to translate this to understandable language for either another health professional or a patient. They also have the interpersonal skills to train other members of staff.

Sales and marketing

Once a drug product is brought to market, the pharmaceutical company will invest a large amount of money on promoting awareness of the product. In the UK, companies are not allowed to market prescription-only medicines directly to the public, although they can market general sales list (GSL) and pharmacy (P) products (under strict guidelines). Adverts for GSL products and 'P' medicines are placed across a range of media outlets, including television, bill boards and magazines.

In addition to this promotion to the general public, companies spend a huge amount of time, money and effort promoting their products to prescribers, who may be doctors, nurses, dentists, pharmacists (more recently) and other health professionals. They also promote their products to the wider pharmacy team that will advise on the prescribing of medicines and make decisions about formularies, both in hospital and community (e.g. primary care trust (PCT) advisory pharmacists). Medical representatives will visit these individuals in their place of work and present the clinical data available on the efficacy and safety of the new product and promote any advantages over the existing products available.

Pharmacists may be involved in developing the marketing of products, and are often involved in focus groups when branding is being developed for a given product. They are also employed as medical representatives where their clinical skills enable them to understand the clinical data involved and to answer complex questions posed by clinicians in relation to the product being marketed. This field represents a relatively small number of pharmacists employed within the pharmaceutical industry.

Regulatory affairs

In the UK the MHRA is the organisation that deals with the licensing and regulation of medicines and medical devices. The MHRA does not have a didactic approach to the enforcement of the regulations surrounding pharmaceutical products. In contrast, the aim of the MHRA is to enable greater access to products, and the timely introduction of innovative treatments and technologies that benefit patients and the public (MHRA, 2007). No product is risk free, and the MHRA makes judgements to ensure that the benefits to patients and the public from these products justify the risks.

As part of this process, the MHRA plays a key role in the regulation of clinical trials (Chamberlain, 2007). Its function is to ensure the safety of trial participants and the collection of valid data. Information must be provided to the MHRA by the pharmaceutical company: the trial protocol, investigators' brochure, inclusion and exclusion criteria, safety monitoring and reporting, non-clinical data and information about the quality of the product and manufacturing conditions (credible data cannot be collected if the quality of a product is inconsistent). The agency does not act in a consultancy role to the sponsoring company. However, it will discuss particular problems that arise during a trial with the company involved.

The MHRA also inspects manufacturing sites of companies and ensures they adhere to GMP guidelines and that the companies facilities are fit for purpose.

When a pharmaceutical company wishes to license a new product for the UK market, once they have completed the appropriate clinical trials, they must submit documentation of various testing performed on the product to the MHRA. This includes a wide range of data collected from in vitro, animal and human studies, data on dosing, indication, pharmacology, pharmacokinetics, routes of elimination, known adverse drug reactions, toxicity, cautions and drug interactions, to name but a few. This must also include specification of purity and acceptable limits for manufacturing of the product (i.e. how must the product perform for it to be deemed 'correct', such as disintegration and dissolution time for a tablet under a given set of experimental conditions). The pharmaceutical company will liaise with the MHRA throughout the process of collecting the clinical data for a product submission, and cooperate towards a (hopefully) successful submission.

The British Pharmacopoeia Commission prepares and publishes the *British Pharmacopoeia* (BP). This book contains monographs for drugs used in the UK in the practice of medicine, surgery, dentistry and midwifery (British Pharmacopoeia Commission, 2007). These monographs contain relevant information (i.e. descriptions of, standards for or notes on other matters relating to these substances). Any medicinal product manufactured or sold in the UK (e.g. by a generics manufacturer) must comply with these standards. The BP also provides guidance on many of the methods that are used to test new drug products for licence submission. Other pharmacopoeias also exist, including the *European Pharmacopoeia*.

Pharmaceutical companies will have a specific department that is responsible for regulatory affairs. This department will collate the large amount of data required for a drug licence submission and transform it into the appropriate format for the particular regulatory agency (depending on the country that registration is being submitted for). This department will also liaise with the different agencies to try to ensure a successful outcome.

Pharmacists are ideally placed to work within these pharmaceutical regulatory bodies and departments. They have the knowledge to be able to interpret both the scientific and clinical data for drugs and to be able to understand the risk–benefit analysis that must be made for all medicines before they can be approved for administration to the public. Equivalent organisations to these UK agencies exist in different countries around the world, for example the Food and Drug Administration (FDA) in the USA. The European Agency for the Evaluation of Medical Products (EMEA) deals with centralised procedures for market authorisations. Opportunities for employment for UK pharmacists also exist in these groups.

General management and business

As with all areas of pharmacy, the different disciplines of industrial pharmacy offer opportunities to move into management. This may involve dealing with staff, economic evaluation of a business situation, budgeting, strategic planning for use of equipment or resources, and critical decision making. Pharmacists are also becoming employed in strategic business roles, facilitating interactions between academia, start-up companies and small and large pharmaceutical companies (Dawson, 1999). The

---

Box 5.3   Case study: Regulatory affairs

As an undergraduate, I did a 6 year course in Pharmaceutical Chemistry and Technology at the University of Trieste, Italy. This course included all the modules of the Pharmacy degree and additional courses relating to the production of pharmaceutical products. My final undergraduate thesis focused on scale-up procedures in granulate production and was carried out in collaboration with a small Italian pharmaceutical company and the University of Bradford in the UK. Whilst at Bradford, I was offered a PhD scholarship sponsored by AstraZeneca to study the stabilising effect of novel excipients on freeze-dried proteins. I conducted my research at the University of Bradford and in AstraZeneca's laboratories in Loughborough in the UK and Södertälje in Sweden. Through my industrial experience, I realised that I enjoyed planning, validating and analysing the experiments and the data collected, rather than the actual running of the experiments.

Whilst writing my PhD thesis, I worked part-time as a locum pharmacist and I started developing an interest in the roles that public bodies such as the National Institute for Health and Clinical Excellence (NICE) and the Medicines and Healthcare products Regulatory Agency (MHRA) have in public health.

Having gained a better understanding of my interests, I came to my current job as a pharmaceutical assessor at the MHRA. As a pharmaceutical assessor, I look at the dossiers of medicines to assess their safety before they get marketing authorisation for the UK and European markets. I work in collaboration with medical doctors and toxicologists and liaise with pharmaceutical companies and other European agencies. In this job, I evaluate all the data collected by pharmaceutical companies in relation to the manufacturing of the product. It is an exciting, stimulating and challenging job that allows me to put into practice what I have learned in my degree and specialised in during my PhD, with the benefit of the perspective I gained during my community experience.

Dr Claudia Vincenzi

Pharmaceutical Assessor, MHRA

multidisciplinary skills of pharmacists make them particularly adept at moving between these different environments.

So you want to be an industrial pharmacist . . . what next?

Undergraduates who are interested in a career in any of the areas of industrial pharmacy should gain relevant work experience. Some companies offer training opportunities to pharmacy students, for example through summer vacation programmes. These can offer an extremely varied experience, depending on the work performed at a particular location, which could range from formulation and analytical testing to clinical trials management and provision of medicines information. Students should enquire about such placements well in advance. Competition for placements is high as only a limited number of companies offer these opportunities; excellent academic performance is vital to getting a placement.

Pre-registration training places within industry are scarce compared with hospital and community pharmacy and thus there is intense competition for placements. However, pre-registration training within this sector is not a prerequisite for a career in industrial pharmacy. Gaining a quality pre-registration placement in another sector, being informed of the different opportunities available in industrial pharmacy and having enthusiasm for work within this sector can be a highly effective route into the industry.

In 2004, 33% of pharmacists working within industrial pharmacy held a PhD (Kerridge, 2004). A further 34% held an additional

---

Box 5.4   Case study: Management and business in pharmaceutical innovation

Although I completed a PhD in Neuropharmacology after getting my degree in Pharmacy, my purpose was not to move into a specific career direction. Embarking on the PhD made me realise that I did not want to become a lecturer or academic researcher. However, during the course of the PhD I came across a programme called Bioscience Young Enterprise Scheme which was open for postgraduate students and which introduced the concept of commercialising science/academic 'know-how'. I participated in this scheme, found it to be very interesting and decided that I wanted to work in this area.

I started out by volunteering my services for 1 month at the newly opened Institute of Pharmaceutical Innovation (IPI) in March 2004. This is a research facility dedicated to supporting innovation in drug development and drug delivery. It performs collaborative research between industry and academia and provides contract services. The IPI had just been opened, so I was seeing a young business operating first hand and found the commercial aspects to be very interesting. I was particularly fortunate as the IPI also enjoyed having me and felt that I was of benefit to the organisation;

I subsequently gained a salaried position and I am still here 3 years later!

My current role is very varied. I have responsibility for developing and maintaining the IPI's marketing materials and website and underpinning the commercialisation and research promotion activity. This involves performing commercial analysis, coordinating agendas for business development and researching new strategic opportunities (e.g. potential new customers, funding initiatives, etc.). I also attend networking events to raise the profile of our capabilities, and organise our conference programme. Other responsibilities include programme management for key commercial projects and start-up companies based within the IPI.

Overall, I enjoy the variety of my role and the fact that my skills and ability can make a real and positive contribution to developing the business and generating revenue for the IPI.

Dr Riddhi Shukla

Commercial Projects Manager, Institute of Pharmaceutical Innovation

qualification relevant to their position (e.g. Qualified Person (QP), Master of Business Administration or a clinical diploma). However, many opportunities exist for training for these qualifications in parallel to employment, supported by an employer. Indeed, industrial pharmacy continues to deliver unparalleled education and career growth opportunities (Wicks, 2000). Certainly qualification and registration with the Royal Pharmaceutical Society of Great Britain, followed by studying for a PhD, is not the only route into this sector of pharmacy. Experience gained after several years of practice in hospital or community pharmacy can be advantageous for some roles within industry (e.g. medicines information, clinical trial supply logistics). There are therefore also opportunities to move into this field a few years after qualification.

Working within the pharmaceutical industry allows you to contribute to the development of new effective and safe medicines benefiting a worldwide population. It presents interesting alternatives that use our professional skills and training, and opportunities to move between different fields and tackle different disciplines of science, information, marketing and management. Most importantly, it presents the chance of an exciting, varied and challenging career.

References

British Pharmacopoeia Commission (2007). *British Pharmacopoeia*. London: Stationery Office.

Chamberlain, J (2007). Legal and regulatory aspects: good control of manufacturing process. *Pharm J* 278: 563–564.

Dawson B. (1999). New challenges: a role for pharmacists in industry. *Pharm J* 263: 534–535.

Kerridge J. (2004). Survey of industrial pharmacists in employment. *Pharm J* 272: 396–397.

Medicines and Healthcare products Regulatory Agency (2007). *How we Regulate*. www.mhra.gov.uk (accessed August 2007).

Proudfoot S (1988). Factors influencing bioavailability: factors influencing drug absorption from the gastrointestinal tract. Pharmaceutics. In: Aulton M, ed. *Pharmaceutics. The Science of Dosage Form Design*. New York: Churchill Livingstone, pp 135–173.

Sharp J (1994). *Quality Rules: Short Guide to Good Manufacturing Practice*, 2nd edn. Reading: Anchor Press.

Wicks S (2000). Careers and development in a growing industrial sector. *Pharm J* 264: 150–151.

Useful resources

RPSBG careers: www.pharmacycareers.org.uk

Association of the British Pharmaceutical Industry (ABPI): www.abpi-careers.org.uk

6

Introduction to medicines management

Rachel L Howard

Introduction

This chapter introduces the concept of medicines management and the role of the community pharmacist. The chapter begins by describing what medicines management is, why it is needed, the different types of medicines management, and how these are achieved. The chapter closes with a description of the medicines management services that community pharmacists in the UK can provide.

Many of the principles of medicines management described in this chapter also apply to hospital pharmacists. However, the specific roles can differ markedly between hospital and community pharmacists; a description of these individual roles is beyond the scope of this chapter.

What is medicines management?

The objective of medicines management is to provide the best possible outcome for patients at the lowest possible cost. Medicines management is not aimed solely at cost reduction, but at providing the most cost-effective care for the best possible patient outcomes. The term medicines management incorporates all aspects of medicines usage by patients and health professionals, including the ways in which medicines are selected, procured, delivered, prescribed, administered, monitored and reviewed. Medicines management has been given a variety of definitions (see Box 6.1), the most succinct of which is, 'the systematic provision of medicines therapy through a partnership effort between patients and professionals to deliver best

---

Box 6.1   Definitions of medicines management

'Medicines management . . . encompasses the entire way that medicines are selected, procured, delivered, prescribed, administered and reviewed to optimise the contribution that medicines make to producing informed and desired outcomes of patient care.' (Audit Commission, 2001)

'Medicines management encompasses a range of activities intended to improve the way that medicines are used, both by patients and by the NHS. Medicines management services are processes based on patient need that are used to design, implement, deliver and monitor patient-focused care. They can include all aspects of the supply and use of medicines, from an individual medication review to a health promotion programme.' (NPC, 2002)

'[Medicines management is a practice that] seeks to maximise health through the optimal use of medicines. It encompasses all aspects of medicines use, from the prescribing of medicines through the ways in which medicines are taken or not taken by patients.' (Lowe, 2001)

'[Medicines management is] the systematic provision of medicines therapy through a partnership of effort between patients and professionals to deliver best patient outcome at minimised cost.' (Tweedie & Jones, 2001)

'[Medicines management is] a pooling of medical, pharmaceutical, and patient knowledge for the benefit of the patient, accessing other professionals' expertise where appropriate.' (Tweedie & Jones, 2001)

---

patient outcome at minimised cost' (Tweedie and Jones, 2001). (Chapter 14 discusses patients and professionals working in partnership.)

Development of medicines management

For many years doctors have been prescribing medicines with the intention of providing patient benefit. Medicines management has not been a focus in the past, so why has there been an increasing emphasis on this area in recent years?

The majority of health professionals and patients recognise that all medicines can cause adverse drug reactions (ADRs). In many cases, these reactions are a minor inconvenience to patients. However, ADRs can result in serious patient injury, leading to hospital admission, disability or even death. These serious ADRs have been studied for many years but, until recently, there has been less interest in whether ADRs could be avoided or the effects on patients lessened. A focus on the preventability of ADRs became apparent in the 1980s with the publication of a number of studies describing

preventable drug-related admissions to hospital (Trunet *et al.*, 1980; Bigby *et al.*, 1987; Italian Group on Intensive Care Evaluation, 1987). In the 1990s the patient safety movement began to gain momentum, with an in-depth analysis of patients' injuries caused by general medical care in US hospitals (Leape *et al.*, 1995). Enthusiasm for maximising the safety, efficacy and quality of patient care reached government level in the UK in 2000 with the publication of the report *An organisation with a memory* (Department of Health, 2000a), which reviewed the literature on medical error and was instrumental in beginning to develop a safety culture in the National Health Service (NHS) (see Box 6.2). In addition, *An organisation with a memory* led to a number of reports highlighting the importance of medicines management and the roles that pharmacists and other health professionals could play (see Boxes 6.3 and 6.4) (Audit Commission, 2001; Smith, 2004). *Pharmacy in the Future* set a deadline of 2004 for the implementation of medicines management schemes in primary care to help 'reduce the amount of illness caused by medicines not being used correctly, and cut waste' (see Box 2.3, page 13) (Department of Health, 2000b).

Box 6.2   An organisation with a memory

An organisation with a memory was a report published by the Department of Health in 2000, in response to a growing recognition of the cost of adverse events within the NHS. It set out:

- what was known about the number and types of adverse events experienced by patients
- where there were holes in our knowledge about the frequency and causes of adverse events
- how other industries, such as aviation and nuclear, have systems in place to learn from mistakes (and therefore help avoid them happening again)
- the role of organisational structures in events leading up to errors, in addition to the role of human errors and the factors which can contribute to these
- the tradition of a 'blame-orientated approach' to individuals when errors occur, whilst advocating

an open and fair approach to individuals which should encourage staff to report adverse events and errors that occur, without fear of retribution
- how existing systems for reporting events are fragmented and incomplete
- a proposal for:

  - a unified national adverse event reporting system allowing analysis of events to help avoid problems in the future
  - a more open culture where errors can be discussed without fear of retribution
  - ensuring that, where lessons are identified, changes are put into place nationally.

The full report can be accessed via www.dh.gov.uk/ en/Publicationsandstatistics/Publications/ PublicationsPolicyAndGuidance/DH_4065083

Box 6.3   A spoonful of sugar

In 2001, the Audit Commission published the report *A spoonful of sugar – medicines management in NHS hospitals* to emphasise the importance of medicines management to managers within National Health Service (NHS) hospitals. The report:

- introduces the concept of medicines management and highlights the obstacles to improving the provision of medicines management
- describes the cost pressures associated with providing medicines for patients and the reasons why medicines management systems should be reviewed
- sets out the medicines management roles of different groups within hospitals, such as hospital managers, drugs and therapeutics

committees, risk managers, clinicians and pharmacists
- highlights ways in which risks can be reduced using computer technology and clinical pharmacists, as well as different ways of providing medicines management
- outlines some of the barriers to an increased role for hospital clinical pharmacists in medicines management, and how these can be overcome
- sets out action plans for managers within NHS hospitals and professional associations in order to improve the provision of medicines management services.

The full report can be accessed via the Audit Commission website (www.audit-commission.gov.uk).

Box 6.4   *Building a safer NHS for patients: improving medication safety*

Following the report *An organisation with a memory* (see Box 6.2), the Department of Health published a series of reports entitled *Building a safer NHS for patients*. One of these – *Improving medication safety* (Smith, 2004) – focused specifically on medication safety. This report described the:

- frequency and causes of medication errors
- role of the National Patient Safety Agency in preventing medication errors
- risks of errors at various stages in the medication use process
- particular risks to patients at high risk of medication errors, such as patients with allergies to medications, seriously ill patients, and children

- risks associated with specific groups of medications
- ways in which medication errors can be avoided through better use of information technology, medication packaging and different ways of working.

The full report can be accessed via www.dh.gov.uk/en/Publicationsandstatistics/Publications/PublicationsPolicyAndGuidance/DH_4071443

National Patient Safety Agency website: www.npsa.nhs.uk

Consequences of poor medicines management

The consequences of poor medicines management include medication errors, patient injury and wastage of NHS money. Medication errors can occur at all stages of the medicines management process (prescribing, dispensing, administering and monitoring). The majority of errors will be identified before the medicines reach patients (near misses) or will result in no harm to patients. However, a significant minority of medication errors (usually those described as serious errors) can result in patient harm (preventable drug-related morbidity; PDRM). The stages of the medicines management process at which errors can occur are described in detail below. The frequency of errors at each stage of the medicines management process is given in Table 6.1.

Table 6.1   Frequency of medication management errors

Error type	Patient group	Frequency of error	Reference
Prescribing error	Children in hospital	0.45–30 errors per 100 prescriptions	Ghaleb *et al.*, 2006
	Adults in hospital	1.5 errors per 100 prescriptions	Dean *et al.*, 2002
	All patients in primary care	0.2–1.9% of prescriptions dispensed in community pharmacy	Chen *et al.*, 2005
Dispensing error	Patients presenting prescriptions to a community pharmacy	22 per 10 000 items dispensed (near misses) 4 per 10 000 items dispensed (errors)	Ashcroft *et al.*, 2005
Administration error	Patients administering their own medication in the community	50% of patients with chronic conditions are poorly adherent	WHO, 2003
	All patients in hospital	15% of patients administered oral medications by nurses	Tissot *et al.*, 2003
		49% of intravenous medication doses administered; one-third of errors at least moderately serious	Taxis and Barber, 2003

Prescribing errors

Prescribing errors can occur when selecting which drug to prescribe, or during the act of writing or computer-generating a prescription. These errors are more frequent in hospitals than in primary care, but still represent a significant risk to patients in the community.

Dispensing errors

Dispensing errors can occur when a medication is physically selected, labelled or handed to the patient. Near misses and dispensing errors are relatively infrequent, but can have important consequences for patients and pharmacists (see Chapter 15). Dispensing errors can cause permanent physical injury or death to patients, and are still considered a criminal offence under the Medicines Act.

Administration errors

Administration errors can occur when a medication is taken by a patient or given to a patient by a carer or health professional. An administration error that results from a patient not taking their medication as prescribed is described as an adherence problem (see Chapter 14). Administration errors can occur when medicines are selected or prepared incorrectly, or administered via the wrong route (see Chapter 16).

Monitoring errors

Both patients and health professionals can make monitoring errors. Monitoring errors can occur when a patient does not recognise that the condition being treated is worsening, or does not act in an appropriate way, such as seeking help from a health professional or adjusting their medication according to a pre-agreed plan. For example, patients with diabetes will find their blood glucose goes up if they have an infection and should therefore be aware of the 'sick day rules', which recommend increasing their insulin dose in response to this. Monitoring errors can also occur when a health professional does not identify a deterioration in a patient's condition, or when they do not perform necessary tests when starting or continuing medication. Tests that health professionals might be expected to perform include blood tests, urine tests and measurement of blood pressure and pulse rate. These can all be used to monitor the effectiveness of medication and to identify potential adverse effects.

Preventable drug-related injuries

Serious medication errors can result in PDRM, which is believed to account for about 4% of admissions to hospital (Howard *et al.*, 2007). Older patients (over 65 years of age) are twice as likely to experience a preventable drug-related admission (Winterstein *et al.*, 2002). Nearly 2% of patients will experience a PDRM during hospital admission (Kanjanarat *et al.*, 2003); in primary care in the USA, 1.5–3% of patients in their own homes, and around 10% of patients in nursing homes, will experience a PDRM (Gurwitz *et al.*, 2000, 2003; Gandhi *et al.*, 2003).

These PDRMs represent a significant burden to patients, health professionals and the NHS. Medication errors are thought to cost the NHS about £500 million per year in extra days spent in hospital. In addition, unused medicines are estimated to waste more than £100 million per year of NHS money (Department of Health, 2000b; Audit Commission, 2001). Improvements to medicines management services in both primary and secondary care settings are an important strategy to help prevent PDRM.

Types of medicines management

Medicines management encompasses a broad range of services that range in focus from individual patients to the provision of care to the population as a whole. Five categories of medicines management services have been identified by the National Prescribing Centre (NPC) and National Primary Care Research & Development Centre (NPCRDC; 2002b):

- clinical medicines management
- systems and processes
- public health
- patients and their medicines
- interface medicines management.

The first four categories are of particular relevance to community pharmacy and are described in more detail below.

Clinical medicines management

Clinical medicines management services focus on the patient and 'the assessment, monitoring and review of prescribing for individual patients' (NPC and NPCRDC, 2002a). All health professionals involved in providing medicines to patients, including pharmacists, have a responsibility to use their clinical and professional skills to provide clinical medicines management services.

In primary care many patients receive medication via repeat prescriptions, which are authorised by the prescriber for a fixed number of prescriptions or a fixed time period (often 6 or 12 months). During this time, the patient requests further prescriptions from the receptionist, rather than making an appointment with their general practitioner (GP). Repeat prescriptions are not checked for their appropriateness each time they are issued. Instead, the prescriptions should be carefully assessed at the end of the repeat prescribing period, a process known as medication review (see Box 6.5). Medication reviews can also be undertaken with patients who are considered to be at a high risk of medication problems, including those taking specific high-risk medications, patients taking more than four regular repeat medications, and patients where poor adherence is suspected (Department of Health, 2001).

Historically, medication reviews have not happened for a variety of reasons, including GPs' time constraints. Zermansky *et al.* (2002) found that GPs performed medication reviews with 56–71% of patients aged 65 years or older on at least one repeat prescription. Guidelines for medication reviews recommend that all patients aged 65 years or older should have an annual medication review, whilst those taking four or more medications should have a medication review every 6 months (Department of Health, 2001). GP practices are now paid for providing medication reviews to patients through the quality and outcomes framework (see Box 2.12) and community pharmacies can be paid for performing medication reviews as an enhanced service in the new community Pharmacy Contract. Medication reviews for patients on repeat prescriptions are an ideal opportunity for pharmacists to contribute to medicines management in primary care. Studies have confirmed that pharmacist-led medication reviews reduce the cost of prescribing, and improve patient adherence to medication (Beney *et al.*, 2000; Holland *et al.*, 2006).

Other clinical medicines management services could include specialist disease management clinics and clinical pharmacy interventions in nursing homes, community hospitals and patients' own homes. Pharmacist-led specialist disease management clinics can improve patients' clinical outcomes, but do not seem to improve the quality of patients' lives (Beney *et al.*, 2000). In addition, the Community Pharmacy Medicines Management Project Evaluation Team (2007) found that although patient satisfaction was increased, community pharmacists had no impact on the appropriateness of drugs prescribed for patients with cardiovascular disease, and the pharmacist-led service cost more than a GP-led service. Thus, the value of any service provided requires serious consideration in terms of patient benefit and cost to the NHS.

Systems and processes

In addition to direct clinical management of patients, some medicines management services focus on the systems and processes of work involved in supplying medicines to patients. The safety and efficiency of medicines management can be improved by changing systems. These medicines management services can include developing protocols for repeat prescribing systems or developing integrated care pathways (flow diagrams that give guidance on how to

Box 6.5   Medication review

Medication review has been defined as, 'a structured critical examination of a patient's medicines, with the objective of reaching an agreement with the patient about treatment, optimising the impact of medicines, minimising the number of medication-related problems and reducing waste' (Shaw *et al.*, 2002). Four different levels of medication review have been identified.

- **Level 0 – *ad hoc*:** An unstructured opportunistic review of a patient's medication in response to a question or problem. *Ad hoc* reviews are not considered to be true medication reviews because they are unlikely to address all of a patient's medication problems.
- **Level 1 – prescription review:** A review of a patient's medication without access to the clinical medical records (see Box 6.7). The patient may not necessarily be present. Prescription reviews can be useful for brand-to-generic switches, deciding whether to continue or discontinue a medicine, and optimising pack sizes. Prescription reviews can also be useful for assessing a patient's medication between face-to-face clinical medication reviews.
- **Level 2 – treatment review:** A review of a patient's medication, often without the patient present, where the reviewer has access to the clinical records. Reviews can cover a patient's whole medication list, or focus on single agents (e.g. lithium, a mood stabiliser used in severe depression, mania and related disorders), or therapeutic groups of agents (e.g.

antihypertensives). Treatment reviews can be used to modify medication doses or to identify patients who need monitoring. Treatment reviews can be problematic because they rely on the treatment record, not the patient's account of what they take, and changes to medication can be made without the patient's agreement. This is not congruent with the concordance model of care (see Chapter 15) and can cause patients to become confused about their medication. This increases the risk of preventable drug-related morbidity through patients mistakenly taking medications incorrectly.

- **Level 3 – clinical medication review (CMR):** A face-to-face review of a patient's medication and clinical condition. A CMR includes a patient's entire medication history (including non-prescription medicines) and takes account of what the patient actually takes and information contained in the medical record. During a CMR, a patient's views and beliefs about their medicines are accounted for and any changes to treatment are agreed with the patient. A CMR facilitates evaluation of the therapeutic value of each drug, identification of untreated conditions, and a concordant discussion about a patient's treatment (see Chapter 15). However, CMRs use a lot of health professional resources (and are therefore more expensive than other reviews). CMRs are considered to be the gold standard, but lower level reviews remain useful for the reasons detailed above.

---

manage patients with specific conditions). In addition, comparing current practice at work with these guidelines or standards (a process known as audit) can help to identify medicines management systems or processes that could be improved (see Chapter 15).

Public health

In addition to focusing medicines management services at individual patients, it is important to target services to meet the needs of the local population – described as public health. Public health services can be targeted at individual members of the public at the point of care, or as part of an educational role within NHS organisations (PSNC, 2004). Medicines management services with a public health focus are shown in Box 6.6. Two of these services are described in more detail below.

Smoking cessation

Community pharmacists can train to provide a successful and cost-effective smoking cessation

Box 6.6   Public health medicines management services

- Smoking cessation
- Coronary heart disease
- Obesity and weight reduction
- Drug misuse (e.g. supervised methadone administration, and needle exchange programmes)
- Sexual health (e.g. provision of emergency hormonal contraception)
- Folic acid and pregnancy
- Asthma (e.g. providing an asthma clinic in conjunction with local GP practices)
- Diabetes (e.g. patient education and monitoring programmes)
- Immunisation (e.g. administering influenza vaccination)
- Head lice (e.g. recommending appropriate treatments such as wet combing)
- Oral health (e.g. encouraging the use of sugar-free medicines in children)

service. Studies in the UK have found that smokers are 2–5-times more likely to quit smoking when they participate in a smoking cessation service led by a community pharmacist (Anderson *et al.*, 2003a).

Influenza vaccination

Community pharmacy patient medication records (PMRs) (see also 'Identifying patients at risk of adverse effects', page 64) can be used to identify patients who might benefit from influenza vaccination (Anderson *et al.*, 2003b). Pharmacists based in supermarket pharmacies in the USA have successfully provided immunisations to adults without adverse effects (Anderson *et al.*, 2003a). A similar service is provided in Scotland where community pharmacists are able to administer influenza vaccination to adults aged 65 years or over as part of a patient group direction: 888 patients were vaccinated through this scheme in 2004 (Hind & Downie, 2006).

Patients and their medicines

As part of the integration of health and social care in the current NHS system (see Chapter 2), some medicines management services also focus on the health and social care aspects of patients and their medicines. Community pharmacies can provide a number of services in this category, including:

- patient education
- medication reviews
- repeat dispensing
- home delivery of medication.

Patient education about medicines should be an integral part of the dispensing process. Increasing patient awareness of how to take their medicines, how to manage potential adverse effects, and how to incorporate their medicine regimens into their daily lives can all be included in patient counselling. In addition, accredited pharmacists working in accredited premises can perform medicines use reviews (see Box 6.7). Domiciliary medication reviews (visiting patients at home or in care homes) can further integrate medicines management with social care. Domiciliary visits provide an ideal opportunity to discuss with patients how they manage their medicines and any problems they may have experienced. A study of older patients in Leeds found that those who had received a domiciliary medication review were more likely to know why they took their medication (Lowe *et al.*, 2000). In addition, patients' medication regimens were simplified and reasons for poor adherence were identified as a result of the medication review.

Ways in which medicines management is achieved

Good medicines management requires all health professionals to develop new skills. In particular, community pharmacists need to develop good working relationships with doctors and patients in order to improve communication with these groups. Good communication is important for a number of reasons.

Box 6.7   Medicines use reviews

Under the new Pharmacy Contract, medicines use reviews (MURs) are an advanced service that can be performed by accredited pharmacists working in accredited community pharmacies. To achieve accreditation, pharmacists must undertake a competency assessment which ensures that they achieve the standards of practice stated in the national competency framework. Training and assessment is provided by various universities (see www.psnc.org.uk for further information). Pharmacy premises require a clearly signposted private consultation area where the pharmacist and patient can sit down and talk at normal speaking volumes without fear of being overheard. Owners of premises complete a self-certification form stating that their premises meet these criteria. This statement is validated by the primary care trust that contracts the service.

MURs provide an opportunity for patients to talk to their community pharmacist about the medicines they are taking, what the medicines do, how well they work, and how to get the most out of them (Department of Health, 2005). In addition, MURs provide the community pharmacist with an opportunity to intervene on prescriptions where they identify problems (Bellingham, 2004). MURs are not a clinical prescription review, and pharmacists do not agree changes to medication with patients – this can only be done by the prescriber. Nor do they discuss patients' medical conditions or the effectiveness of their treatment on the basis of test results (PSNC, 2007a). Community pharmacists should agree an action plan with patients which is then communicated to the appropriate health professional(s), who might include the general practitioner, practice nurse, community matron, prescribing pharmacist or district nurse.

By February 2007, 13 611 pharmacists had been accredited and in November 2006, 63 455 MURs were conducted in 4167 accredited community pharmacies in England (PSNC, 2007b). In 2007/8, pharmacies were paid £25 for each MUR.

- If community pharmacists are to advise doctors and other prescribers on medicines issues for individual patients, or on systems of medicines management, they must learn how to communicate confidently but diplomatically.
- If community pharmacists are to help patients manage their medicines effectively, then they must develop good listening skills and learn to move away from a compliance model of practice (where patients are expected to do as they are told) to a concordance model (where patients are supported by health professionals to choose the treatment options most appropriate for them). More information on compliance and concordance is provided in Chapter 14.
- In addition, community pharmacists need to develop a good understanding of the risks associated with the medications they supply, to help them identify inappropriate prescriptions and over-the-counter sales.

Communication with patients

Lack of communication skills has been identified as a barrier to community pharmacists providing medicines management services in the UK (Van Mil *et al.*, 2001). Studies conducted in the UK found that older patients only had contact with a community pharmacist on 12.5–15% of the times they collected a prescription from a pharmacy (Livingstone, 1996; Jones *et al.*, 1997). In addition, community pharmacists have historically spent a limited amount of time talking to patients about their medicines, the mean contact time for patient counselling ranging from 20 seconds to just over a minute (Savage, 1995; Livingstone, 1996). If pharmacists are to provide effective medicines management services, they need to spend more time talking to patients about their medicines. The new Pharmacy Contract encourages increased contact time with patients by paying community pharmacists for providing medicines use reviews (see Box 6.7). This service helps pharmacists to provide a structured discussion with patients about their medicines and will hopefully help to overcome some of the barriers to communicating with patients, such as time and workload pressures (Savage, 1995; Smith *et al.*, 2004), lack of remuneration (Anderson *et al.*, 2003c), lack of training (Anderson *et al.*, 2003c), and lack of privacy (Sleath, 1996). Under the new Pharmacy Contract, pharmacists providing medicines use reviews are required to have a private consultation room, which should help to ensure patient privacy. Communication with patients is described in more detail in Chapter 8.

Communication with health professionals

In addition to developing good relationships with patients, it is important that community pharmacists develop good relationships with other health professionals, particularly GPs and other prescribers. This is essential to ensure that they can effectively intervene on high-risk prescriptions, and act as a source of information to prescribers about medicines and their use. It is important to remember that many community pharmacists play a vital role in preventing prescribing errors from reaching patients. The better a community pharmacist's communication skills, the more effective they are likely to be in this role.

Pharmacists may be reluctant to contact GPs about prescriptions that may cause a patient harm because: they lack confidence in their knowledge about the medication; they do not have access to the patient's medical records (and therefore do not understand the bigger picture of the patient's treatment); they have previously had their advice ignored when they have contacted a GP (Moody *et al.*, 2004); they have found GPs to be aggressive, rude or unapproachable (Landers *et al.*, 2002; Howard *et al.*, 2008). In addition, some pharmacists believe that GPs view them as subordinate, which may lead some community pharmacists to communicate with GPs in a deferential manner (Hughes and McCann, 2003), an approach that is unlikely to prove effective when wanting to get a prescription changed (Chen *et al.*, 1999).

Hawksworth *et al.* (1999) found that nearly one-fifth of recommendations made by community pharmacists to GPs were rejected. In one case, had the intervention been accepted, it would almost certainly have helped avoid a hospital admission. Considering how infrequently community pharmacists contact GPs to make interventions (only 75 interventions per 10 000 prescriptions dispensed), pharmacists should develop the skills necessary to maximise the impact of the interventions they do make. In addition, community pharmacists need clinical knowledge about medicines, which will help them to intervene on prescriptions more frequently. (See Chapter 15 for examples of the consequences for pharmacists when they do not intervene on prescriptions that cause a patient harm.)

In essence, community pharmacists need to build relationships with GPs and other prescribers wherever possible, in order to increase their effectiveness when making interventions on prescriptions. Face-to-face meetings (perhaps to discuss ways in which pharmacists and GPs can work more closely together and to increase GPs' understanding of the role of the community pharmacist) have been found to improve trust and communication between community pharmacists and GPs (Chen *et al.*, 2001; Zillich *et al.*, 2005). In particular, face-to-face meetings can improve pharmacists' confidence when they talk to GPs. This should help to avoid situations in which pharmacists use a deferential approach or GPs are dismissive of their recommendations.

Identifying patients at risk of adverse effects

As a profession, pharmacists promote themselves on the basis of their specialist knowledge about medicines; however, there is some evidence that they do not always apply this knowledge (Harding & Taylor, 1997). In order to perform an effective medicines management service, it is essential that community pharmacists have a robust understanding of the risks associated with the medications that they supply, and develop the skills necessary to identify when patients are at risk of PDRM. Community pharmacists' knowledge about medication may be insufficient for a number of reasons.

Some community pharmacists may have difficulty accessing training (Howard, 2006) and this may contribute to their varying levels of commitment to continuing professional development (CPD) (Attewell *et al.*, 2005). In addition, some pharmacies may not provide access to appropriate information resources such as the electronic *British National Formulary*, online datasheets or *Stockley's Drug Interactions* (Howard, 2006). Most pharmacists have limited access to patients' medical records and rely on the PMR for a medication history. PMRs are often incomplete because they rarely include over-the-counter medications and rely on patients attending the same pharmacy each time a prescription is dispensed (whereas patients will often attend the most convenient pharmacy). This lack of access to patient-specific information can make it particularly difficult for a community pharmacist to assess the appropriateness of new and ongoing medications.

Pharmacists do, however, have access to quite a lot of patient-specific information including:

- **patient age:** prescriptions for children and older patients should be scrutinised carefully because they are at a higher risk of experiencing adverse effects
- **prescription exemptions:** patients with diabetes, renal dialysis, Addison's disease, myasthenia gravis, epilepsy, hypothyroidism will have an exemption form stating that they have a medical exemption; individual patients will have to be asked what the exemption is for
- **pregnancy and breastfeeding** patients will have a maternity exemption certificate which is valid from the date of issue to 12 months after the date of birth
- **PMR:** although the PMR may be incomplete, it can still provide a useful guide to concurrent medication for patients who regularly attend the same pharmacy. It can help pharmacists to identify inappropriate changes in medication dose, drug interactions and contraindicated drugs (based on drug treatments for specific diseases, e.g. patients prescribed inhalers could have asthma)

- **Patient or relative:** patients will often be able to tell you if they take medicines that have a high risk of interaction with other medicines, such as warfarin (an anticoagulant).

This information should be taken into account when assessing the appropriateness of a prescription. If a pharmacist identifies a prescription that may cause harm to the patient, they should contact the prescriber to clarify whether the patient is at risk, and, if this risk is unacceptable, request that the prescription is changed.

Pharmacists should keep a record of any recommendations they make. This record can be used to audit the provision of medicines management services (with a view to improving the services), to assess the appropriateness of recommendations, and to help pharmacists reflect on their recommendations and identify any areas where their knowledge base is weak. This can form part of their CPD cycle (see Chapter 15).

Community pharmacists and medicines management under the new Pharmacy Contract

The new Pharmacy Contract for the supply of services to the NHS by community pharmacists was introduced in England and Wales in 2005. This contract introduced three tiers of service provision:

- essential (Box 6.8)
- advanced (medicines use reviews and prescription interventions; Box 6.7)
- enhanced (Box 6.9).

Essential services have to be provided by all NHS pharmacy contractors in England and Wales, whilst advanced services can only be provided by accredited contractors. In addition, the enhanced services are provided on the basis of local need. This means that only the services that local primary care trusts (PCTs) buy (commonly known as commissioning) are provided. It is not enough, however, for pharmacists to wait for PCTs to commission these services. In the new competitive market

---

Box 6.8   Essential services

- **Dispensing:** 'medicines and appliances ordered on NHS prescriptions together with information and advice to enable safe and effective use by patients and carers and maintenance of appropriate records.' (PSNC 2004b)
- **Repeat dispensing:** 'management and dispensing of repeatable NHS prescriptions for medicines and appliances in partnership with the patient and the prescriber. . . Ascertain[ing] the patient's need for a repeat supply and communicat[ing] any clinically significant issues to the prescriber.' (PSNC 2004e)
- **Disposing of unwanted medicines:** 'Acceptance by community pharmacies of unwanted medicines from households and individuals which require safe disposal.' (PSNC 2004c)
- **Promoting healthy lifestyles (Public Health):** Providing 'opportunistic advice on lifestyle and public health issues to patients receiving prescriptions. . . [pro-actively participating] in national/local campaigns to promote public health messages to general pharmacy visitors during

specific targeted campaign periods.' (PSNC 2004d)
- **Signposting:** Providing 'information to people visiting the pharmacy who require further support, advice or treatment which cannot be provided by the pharmacy on other health and social care providers or support organisations who may be able to assist the person' including referrals to other health or social care providers, if appropriate. (PSNC 2004f)
- **Support for self-care:** Providing advice and support 'to enable people to derive maximum benefit from caring for themselves or their families.' (PSNC 2004g)
- **Clinical governance:** 'Identify a clinical governance lead and apply the principles of clinical governance (see Chapter 16) to the delivery of services in the pharmacy including standard operating procedures; recording, reporting and learning from adverse incidents; participation in continuing professional development and clinical audit; and assessing patient satisfaction.' (PSNC 2004a)

---

of the NHS, community pharmacists need to actively identify local service needs and campaign the PCTs to ensure that these services are commissioned from community pharmacies. Community pharmacists can identify the service needs of their local population in numerous ways.

- **Discussion with PCTs:** Each PCT will have a 'commissioner', the person who is responsible for buying in services. In addition, medicines management teams (including the prescribing adviser and practice pharmacists) will have identified local medicines management needs. Community pharmacists can offer to provide some of these services.
- **National Service Frameworks (NSFs):** The Government has published a series of guidelines for managing specific patient groups such as older people and children. The NSFs include a number of enhanced services that could be provided by community pharma-

cists, for example clinical medication reviews.
- **Local patient prospectus:** This describes where NHS funds have been spent and which services are offered locally, and can be useful to help identify gaps in local service provision.
- **Local knowledge:** Community pharmacists have regular contact with the general public in their local area. This allows them to build a picture of their patient group, and the types of services they most need.
- **Patient feedback on services:** This can be gained formally (through questionnaires) or informally through comments made by patients when you talk to them. Patient feedback can be used to evaluate existing services, and to identify which services the general public would like to be provided.

Armed with the above information about existing services and service needs in the local population, community pharmacists can approach the commissioners within the local PCT to propose

---

Box 6.9   Enhanced services

- **Supervised administration:** Supervise 'the consumption of prescribed medicines at the point of dispensing in the pharmacy, ensuring that the dose has been administered to the patient, [as part of a] user-friendly, non-judgmental, client-centred and confidential service' , for example for methadone, and medicines used for the management of mental health conditions or tuberculosis (PSNC, 2005h).

- **Needle and syringe exchange:** 'provide access to sterile needles and syringes, and sharps containers for return of used equipment. Where agreed locally, associated materials, for example condoms, citric acid and swabs, to promote safe injecting practice and reduce transmission of infections by substance misusers will be provided.' Appropriate public health education will also be provided to service users. (PSNC, 2005g)

- **Smoking cessation:** 'provide one-to-one support and advice to smokers, refer to specialist services if necessary, and facilitate access to, and where appropriate supply, appropriate stop smoking drugs and aids.' (PSNC, 2005g)

- **Care home (support and advice on storage, supply and administration of drugs and appliances):** 'ensure the proper and effective ordering of drugs and appliances and their clinical and cost effective use, their safe storage, supply and administration and proper record keeping in care homes such as nursing and residential homes.' (PSNC, 2005a)

- **Medicines Assessment & Compliance Support:** 'Medicines support over and above that provided as part of the essential and enhanced services, including assessment of patients' ability to take their medicines and the supply of compliance aids as appropriate, including compliance charts, screw top closures, medication administration record (MAR) charts, labelling medicines in large fonts and multi-compartment compliance aids.' (PSNC, 2005d)

- **Full (level 3) clinical medication review** (see Box 6.5) (PSNC, 2005c)

- **Minor ailment service:** Providing 'advice and support to people on the management of minor ailments, including where necessary, the supply of medicines for the treatment of the minor ailment, for those people who would have otherwise gone to their GP for a prescription.' (PSNC, 2005e)

- **Out-of-hours service:** 'Providing access to pharmacy services during an extended period of opening to ensure that people have prompt access to medicines during the out of hours period.' (PSNC, 2005f)

- **Supplementary prescribing:** 'Implementing patient specific clinical management plans (CMP) with the patient's and doctor's agreement, including prescribing medicines, ordering diagnostic tests, monitoring test results and response to treatment, adjusting treatment accordingly, and referring to other primary healthcare professionals as appropriate.' (PSNC, 2005i)

- **Emergency Hormonal Contraception Service:** 'Providing, free of charge, levonorgestrel emergency hormonal contraception (EHC) to customers within the constraints of a patient group direction (PGD). If customers requesting EHC fall outside the PGD, they should be referred to an appropriate healthcare professional or sold the product OTC (if appropriate). All customers requesting EHC should be given appropriate counselling about contraception and sexually transmitted infections.' (PSNC, 2005b)

---

new services that could be provided (which the PCT can then pay for). For example, Lloyds Pharmacy in London now offers a 'stop now' service and a 'cut down and quit' service for smokers, which include free weekly consultations where carbon monoxide readings are taken and advice is given on managing withdrawal symptoms (Pharmaceutical Journal, 2007).

The new Pharmacy Contract has begun a shift in the source of funding for community pharmacy services away from dispensing large volumes of prescriptions. By providing funding to pharmacies for wider medicines management services, the aim is to expand the role of community pharmacists in providing health and social care services to the general public.

Summary

Medicines management has arisen from the recognition that drugs can cause injury to patients, but that many of these injuries are potentially preventable if services for managing medicines are improved. In the UK, medicines management aims to deliver the best possible outcomes for patients whilst minimising cost to the NHS. It is not simply about cost cutting, but about cost-effectiveness.

Medicines management is a complex process, involving various stages in medication use (prescribing, dispensing, administering and monitoring) and multiple people, including a range of health professionals, patients and their carers. Medicines management services have been divided into five categories: clinical, systems and processes, public health, patients and their medicines, and interface management.

Provision of good medicines management services requires community pharmacists to build relationships with both patients and prescribers. To do this, they need to develop excellent communication skills and ensure they have a good understanding of the risks associated with the medicines they supply. In addition, they must develop the necessary skills to identify patients at risk from medicines management problems, such as problems adhering to medicines, and potential drug interactions or contraindicated medicines.

The new Pharmacy Contract has provided community pharmacists with a different way of funding their work, which should encourage them to provide a broader range of medicines management services.

References

Anderson C, Blenkinsopp A, Armstrong M (2003a). *The contribution of community pharmacy to improving the public's health. Report 1: Evidence from the peer-reviewed literature 1990–2001*. London: Pharmacy Health Link.

Anderson C, Blenkinsopp A, Armstrong M (2003b). *The contribution of community pharmacy to improving the public's health. Report 2: Evidence from the UK non peer-reviewed literature 1990–2002*. London: Pharmacy Health Link.

Anderson C, Blenkinsopp A, Armstrong M (2003c). Pharmacists' perceptions regarding their contribution to improving the public's health: A systematic review of the United Kingdom and international literature 1990–2001. *Int J Pharm Pract* 11: 111–120.

Ashcroft D M, Quinlan P, Blenkinsopp A (2005). Prospective study of the incidence, nature and causes of dispensing errors in community pharmacies. *Pharmacoepidemiol Drug Saf* 14: 327–332.

Attewell J, Blenkinsopp A, Black P (2005). Community pharmacists and continuing professional development – A qualitative study of perceptions and current involvement. *Pharm J* 247: 519–524.

Audit Commission (2001). *A spoonful of sugar – Medicines Management in NHS hospitals*. www.audit-commission.gov.uk/Products/NATIONAL-REPORT/E83C8921–6CEA-4b2c-83E7–F80954A80F85/nrspoonfulsugar.pdf.

Bellingham C (2004). How to offer a medicines use review. *Pharm J* 273: 602.

Beney J, Bero L A, Bond C (2000). Expanding the roles of outpatient pharmacists: effects on health services utilisation, costs, and patient outcomes. *Cochrane Database Syst Rev,* issue 2, CD000336.

Bigby J, Dunn J, Goldman L, *et al.* (1987). Assessing the preventability of emergency hospital admissions. A method for evaluating the quality of medical care in a primary care facility. *Am J Med* 83: 1031–1036.

Chen T F, Crampton M, Krass I, *et al.* (1999). Collaboration between community pharmacists and GPs – the medication review process. *J Soc Admin Pharm* 16: 145–156.

Chen T F, Crampton M, Krass I, *et al.* (2001). Collaboration between community pharmacists and GPs – impact on interprofessional communication. *J Soc Admin Pharm* 18: 83–90.

Chen Y F, Neil K E, Avery A J, *et al.* (2005). Prescribing errors and other problems reported by community pharmacists. *Ther Clin Risk Manage* 1: 333–342.

Community Pharmacy Medicines Management Project Evaluation Team (2007). The MEDMAN study: a randomized controlled trial of community pharmacy-led medicines management for patients with coronary heart disease. *Fam Pract* 24: 189–200.

Dean B, Schachter M, Vincent C, *et al.* (2002). Prescribing errors in hospital inpatients: their incidence and clinical significance. *Qual Saf Health Care* 11: 340–344.

Department of Health (2000a). *An Organisation with a Memory.* www.dh.gov.uk/en/Publicationsandstatistics/Publications/PublicationsPolicyAndGuidance/DH_4065083.

Department of Health (2000b). *Pharmacy in the Future – Implementing the NHS Plan. A programme for pharmacy in the National Health Service.* www.dh.gov.uk/en/Publicationsandstatistics/Publications/PublicationsPolicyAndGuidance/DH_4005917.

Department of Health (2001). *Medicines for older people: Implementing medicines-related aspects of the NSF for older people.* www.dh.gov.uk/en/Publicationsandstatistics/Publications/PublicationsPolicyAndGuidance/DH_4008020.

Department of Health (2005). *Medicines use review: Understand your medicines.* www.dh.gov.uk/en/Publicationsandstatistics/Publications/PublicationsPolicyAndGuidance/DH_4126843 (accessed 20 December 2007).

Gandhi T K, Weingart S N, Borus J, *et al.* (2003). Adverse drug events in ambulatory care. *New Engl J Med* 348: 1556–1564.

Ghaleb M A, Barber N, Franklin B D, *et al.* (2006). Systematic review of medication errors in pediatric patients. *Ann Pharmacother* 40: 1766–76.

Gurwitz J H, Field T S, Avorn J, *et al.* (2000). Incidence and preventability of adverse drug events in nursing homes. *Am J Med* 109: 87–94.

Gurwitz J H, Field T S, Harrold L R, *et al.* (2003). Incidence and preventability of adverse drug events among older persons in the ambulatory setting. *J Am Med Assoc* 289: 1107–16.

Harding G, Taylor K (1997). Responding to change: the case of community pharmacy in Great Britain. *Sociol Health Illn* 19: 547–560.

Hawksworth G M, Corlett A J, Wright D J, *et al.* (1999). Clinical pharmacy interventions by community pharmacists during the dispensing process. *Br J Clin Pharmacol* 47: 695–700.

Hind C, Downie G (2006). Vaccine administration in pharmacies – a Scottish success story. *Pharm J* 277: 134–136.

Holland R, Smith R, Harvey I (2006). Where now for pharmacist led medication review? *J Epidemiol Community Health* 60: 92–93.

Howard R L (2006). The underlying causes of preventable drug-related admissions to hospital. [PhD thesis]. University of Nottingham.

Howard R L, Avery A J, Slavenburg S, *et al.* (2007). Which drugs cause preventable admissions to hospital? A systematic review. *Br J Clin Pharmacol* 63: 136–147.

Howard R L, Avery A J, Bissell P (2008). The underlying causes of preventable drug-related hospital admissions: a qualitative study. *Qual Saf Health Care,* in press.

Hughes C M, McCann S (2003). Perceived interprofessional barriers between community pharmacists and general practitioners: a qualitative assessment. *Br J Gen Pract* 53: 600–606.

Italian Group on Intensive Care Evaluation (1987). Epidemiology of adverse drug reactions in intensive care units. A multicentre prospective study. *Eur J Clin Pharmacol* 31: 507–512.

Jones D, Seymour R, Woodhouse K (1997). Use of pharmacists by older people in the community. *Arch Gerontol Geriatr* 24: 9–13.

Kanjanarat P, Winterstein A G, Johns T E, *et al.* (2003). Nature of preventable adverse drug events in hospitals: A literature review. *Am J Health Syst Pharm* 60: 1750–1759.

Landers M, Blenkinsopp A, Pollock K, *et al.* (2002). Community pharmacists and depression: the pharmacist as intermediary between patient and physician. *Int J Pharm Pract* 10: 253–265.

Leape L L, Bates D W, Cullen D J, *et al.* (1995). Systems analysis of adverse drug events. ADE Prevention Study Group. *J Am Med Assoc* 274: 35–43.

Livingstone C (1996). Verbal interactions between elderly people and community pharmacists about prescription medicines. *Int J Pharm Pract* 4: 12–18.

Lowe C (2001). What medicines management means. *Pharm J* 267: 206–207.

Lowe C J, Raynor D K, Purvis J, *et al.* (2000). Effects of a medicine review and education programme for older people in general practice. *Br J Clin Pharmacol* 50: 172–5.

Moody M, Hansford D, Blake L, *et al.* (2004). Would community pharmacists welcome electronic access to patients' clinical data? *Pharm J* 272: 94–97.

NPC (2002). Medicines management services – why are they so important? *MeReC Bull* 12: 21–23.

NPC, NPCRDC (2002a). *Modernising Medicines Management. A guide to achieving benefits for patients, professionals and the NHS (Book 1).* Liverpool: National Prescribing Centre. www.npc.co.uk/publications/mmm_guide_1.pdf.

NPC, NPCRDC (2002b). *Modernising Medicines Management. A guide to achieving benefits for patients, professionals and the NHS (Book 2).* Liverpool: National Prescribing Centre. Available from http://www.npc.co.uk/publications/mmm_guide_2.pdf.

PSNC (2007a). *Medicines Use Review: What GPs and practice managers need to know.* Available via www.psnc.org.uk (accessed 1 March 2007)

PSNC (2007b). *MUR statistics.* www.psnc.org.uk/index.php?type=page&pid=72&k=3 (accessed 1 March 2007).

Pharmaceutical Journal (2007). Flint launches Lloyds pharmacy smoking cessation campaign. *Pharm J* 278: 698.

PSNC (2004a). *Essential Service – Clinical governance*

requirements in the new community pharmacy contractual framework. Available via www.psnc.org.uk

PSNC (2004b). *NHS Community Pharmacy Contractual Framework. Essential Service – Dispensing.* Available via www.psnc.org.uk

PSNC (2004c). *NHS Community Pharmacy Contractual Framework. Essential Service – Disposal of unwanted medicines.* Available via www.psnc.org.uk

PSNC (2004d). *NHS Community Pharmacy Contractual Framework. Essential Service – Promotion of healthy lifestyles (Public Health).* Available via www.psnc.org.uk

PSNC (2004e). *NHS Community Pharmacy Contractual Framework. Essential Service – Repeat Dispensing.* Available via www.psnc.org.uk

PSNC (2004f). *NHS Community Pharmacy Contractual Framework. Essential Service – Signposting.* Available via www.psnc.org.uk

PSNC (2004g). *NHS Community Pharmacy Contractual Framework. Essential Service – Support for self-care.* Available via www.psnc.org.uk

PSNC, *et al.* (2004). *Public Health: a practical guide for community pharmacists.* London, Pharmacy Health Link. Available from www.pharmacyhealthlink.org.uk

PSNC (2005a). *NHS Community Pharmacy Contractual Framework. Enhanced Service – Care Home (support and advice on storage, supply and administration of drugs and appliances).* Available via www.psnc.org.uk

PSNC (2005b). *NHS Community Pharmacy Contractual Framework. Enhanced Service – Emergency Hormonal Contraception Service.* Available via www.psnc.org.uk

PSNC (2005c). *NHS Community Pharmacy Contractual Framework. Enhanced Service – Medication Review (Full Clinical Review).* Available via www.psnc.org.uk

PSNC (2005d). *NHS Community Pharmacy Contractual Framework. Enhanced Service – Medicines Assessment & Compliance Support.* Available via www.psnc. org.uk

PSNC (2005e). *NHS Community Pharmacy Contractual Framework. Enhanced Service – Minor Ailment Service.* Available via www.psnc.org.uk

PSNC (2005f). *NHS Community Pharmacy Contractual Framework. Enhanced Service – Out of Hours (Access to Medicines).* Available via www.psnc.org.uk

PSNC (2005g). *NHS Community Pharmacy Contractual Framework. Enhanced Service – Stop Smoking.* Available via www.psnc.org.uk

PSNC (2005h). *NHS Community Pharmacy Contractual Framework. Enhanced Service – Supervised Administration (Consumption of Prescribed Medicines).* Available via www.psnc.org.uk

PSNC (2005i). *NHS Community Pharmacy Contractual Framework. Enhanced Service – Supplementary Prescribing by Pharmacists.* Available via www.psnc.org.uk.

Savage I T (1995). Time for customer contact in pharmacies with and without a dispensing technician. *Int J Pharm Pract* 3: 193–199.

Shaw J, Seal R, Pilling M (2002). *Room for Review: a Guide to Medication Review.* www.npc.co.uk/med%5Fpartnership/medication-review/room-for-review.

Sleath B (1996). Pharmacist-patient relationships: authoritarian, participatory, or default? *Patient Educ Couns* 28: 253–263.

Smith J (2004). *Building a safer NHS for Patients: Improving Medication Safety.* London, Department of Health. www.dh.gov.uk/en/Publicationsandstatistics/Publications/PublicationsPolicyAndGuidance/DH_4071443.

Smith S R, Golin C E, Reif S (2004). Influence of time stress and other variables on counselling by pharmacists about antiretroviral medications. *Am J Health Syst Pharm* 61: 1120–1129.

Taxis K, Barber N (2003). Causes of intravenous medication errors: an ethnographic study. *Qual Saf Health Care* 12: 343–348.

Tissot E, Cornette C, Limat S, *et al.* (2003). Observational study of potential risk factors of medication administration errors. *Pharm World Sci* 25: 264–268.

Trunet P, Le Gall J R, Lhoste F, *et al.* (1980). The role of iatrogenic disease in admissions to intensive care. *J Am Med Assoc* 244: 2617–2620.

Tweedie A, Jones I (2001). What is medicines management? *Pharm J* 266: 248.

Van Mil J W F, De Boer W O, Tromp T F J (2001). European barriers to the implementation of pharmaceutical care. *Int J Pharm Pract* 9: 163–168.

Winterstein A G, Sauer B C, Hepler C D, *et al.* (2002). Preventable drug-related hospital admissions. *Ann Pharmacother* 36: 1238–1248.

World Health Organization (2003). *Adherence to long-term therapies. Evidence for action.* Geneva: WHO.

Zermansky A G, Petty D R, Raynor D K, *et al.* (2002). Clinical medication review by a pharmacist of patients on repeat prescriptions in general practice: a randomised controlled trial. *Health Technol Assess* 6: 1–86.

Zillich A J, Doucette W R, Carter B L, *et al.* (2005). Development and initial validation of an instrument to measure physician-pharmacist collaboration from the physician perspective. *Value Health* 8: 59–66.

7

Structure and function of the Royal Pharmaceutical Society of Great Britain

Kate E Fletcher

Introduction

This chapter describes the structure and function of the Royal Pharmaceutical Society of Great Britain (RPSGB) at the time of writing (late 2007). However, The Health Act 1999 may result in fundamental changes to the regulation of health professions and health professionals. This is likely to include pharmacists and the role of the RPSGB. Such changes have not yet been announced or formalised. A detailed description of the history and structure of the RPSGB can be found on their website www.rpsgb.org/societyfunctions/aboutthesociety, from which information in this chapter is taken.

The Royal Pharmaceutical Society of Great Britain

The RPSGB is the professional and regulatory body for pharmacists in England, Scotland and Wales. In order to practise as a pharmacist in these countries, an individual must be registered on the Register of Pharmaceutical Chemists. Entry on to the Register is controlled by the RPSGB.

To qualify for registration, an individual must have completed a 4 year masters degree in pharmacy from one of the 23 Schools of Pharmacy, completed 12 months' pre-registration work-based training, and passed the registration examination. A fee is payable to be added to the register, and an annual retention fee to remain on the register. Pharmacists who gained their qualifications in other countries may be eligible for registration with the RPSGB, although many of these individuals will have to undertake further study, examination and training to meet the standards for registration.

The primary objectives of the RPSGB are to lead, regulate, develop and represent the profession of pharmacy. The Society also works to advance science, practice, education and knowledge in pharmacy, and to promote the profession to external stakeholders, such as the Department of Health.

The Society is also responsible for assuring the competence and fitness to practise of those on the register. It uses various means to achieve this, including:

- controlling entry on to the register
- regulating and accrediting undergraduate pharmacy degrees
- setting and enforcing professional standards
- promoting good practice
- dealing with poor performance and providing support for improvement
- dealing with misconduct and removal from the register.

Indeed, the combined role of representation and regulation of pharmacists makes the RPSGB unique amongst similar bodies in the UK. Other health professions are represented and regulated by separate organisations (see The Future of the RPSGB on page 74).

The *Pharmaceutical Journal*

The Society has published the *Pharmaceutical Journal* since 1841. 'The PJ', as it is often known, is the official journal of the Society. It has been published weekly since 1870, and aims to provide comprehensive news coverage on all aspects of pharmacy and to publish original research and articles on pharmaceutical and related subjects. It is also the main publication in which jobs for pharmacists and pharmacy technicians are advertised. More about the *Pharmaceutical Journal* can be found at www.pjonline.com.

A brief history of the Society

For thousands of years, humans have harnessed the properties of plants and naturally occurring compounds in an attempt to treat illness (see Chapter 3). Over time, the people involved in this process became more specialised, and recognised as skilled individuals. By the 18th century, the terms chemist and druggist were being used in the UK to describe the (mainly) men who compounded medicines. The term used today for this profession is pharmacist.

Pharmacy as a profession was unregulated and unprotected for many years, until the early 19th century, when some chemists and druggists began working together to protect the profession's interests. They argued for an exemption from the Apothecaries Act of 1815, which threatened to restrict the work of chemists and druggists. The act recognised apothecaries as medical practitioners, and gave them certain power over others. Unqualified persons were forbidden to act or practise as apothecaries, and faced a penalty of £20 if they did so. This act therefore threatened the livelihood of chemists and druggists. The group also formed a committee to monitor progress of a proposed Sale of Poisons Bill in 1819, and created a short-lived General Association of Chemists and Druggists to protect them against the Medicine Stamp Act. This act required a duty stamp to be fixed to the packaging of manufactured medicines that were not deemed to be of a standard well-known recipe. The tax paid was in proportion to the cost of the medicine. On a shilling (12 penny) remedy it would be one and a half pence (Homan, 2002).

In 1841, the profession felt vulnerable; it was unregulated and unrestricted, so anyone could use the title of chemist and/or druggist. On 15 April of that year, a group of eminent chemists and druggists met at the *Crown and Anchor Tavern* in the Strand, London. Their aim was to unite the profession into one body, to protect its members' interests and advance scientific knowledge. The group agreed the best foundation for a permanent independent association was membership based on a recognised qualification. William Allen proposed the formation of the Pharmaceutical Society. He went on to become the Society's first president. A committee of 40 was appointed as the first council to frame laws and regulations. This was superseded in May 1842 by an elected council of 21 members. The Society took up residence in 17 Bloomsbury Square in September 1841, where it remained until the new headquarters in Lambeth, South London, were opened in September 1976.

The Society gained its Royal Charter of Incorporation from Queen Victoria in 1843. A charter is an authority directly from the monarch for a body to take certain powers (Appelbe & Wingfield, 2005). A Charter of Incorporation enables a body to function as a corporation (i.e. a large company or group of companies authorised to act as a single entity and recognised as such in law). The Charter gave precedence to 'advancing chemistry and pharmacy and promoting a uniform system of education' over 'the protection of those who carry on the business of chemists and druggists' (The Royal Charter of Incorporation, 1843). The charter also gave the Society a corporate framework that has been refined by supplemental charters in 1901, 1948, 1953 and 2004.

King George VI became the Society's patron in March 1937, and the monarch has been the patron of the Society ever since. Queen Elizabeth II granted the title 'Royal' to the Society in May 1988.

The structure of the RPSGB

The Royal Pharmaceutical Council

The Royal Pharmaceutical Council governs the RPSGB and is responsible for deciding policy and practice relating to the RPSGB. It is composed of:

- 17 pharmacists, elected by the membership of the Society by postal single transferable vote
- 1 pharmacist appointed by universities awarding pharmacy degrees accredited by the Society
- 2 elected pharmacy technicians (elected by technicians on the voluntary register of pharmacy technicians)
- 10 lay members appointed by the Privy Council.

The Council elects its own President.

The purpose of the supplemental charter of 2004 was essentially to modernise the charter of 1953 and make it fit for the purpose of enabling the Society to function in the 21st century. One result of the charter was to alter the tenure of council members: members elected after the supplemental charter of 2004 came into force

serve for terms of 1, 2 or 3 years, allocated according to the number of votes received. Before this elected members were appointed for a 3 year period.

The Council meets six times a year. It is advised on specialist areas of pharmacy by committees and subcommittees, membership and special interest groups. Examples include the Education Committee, Practice Committee, Science Committee, Community Pharmacists Group, Hospital Pharmacists Group and the Industrial Pharmacists Group.

The Committees of the RPSGB

The RPSGB exercises is powers through nine committees.

- **The Education Committee** is responsible for setting educational standards and accrediting providers. It covers undergraduate education, pre-registration training, continuing professional development (CPD) and pharmacy technician education.
- **The Law and Ethics Committee** implements policy relating to professional conduct and the legal aspects of pharmacy practice.
- **The Science Committee** is responsible for implementing science policy; considers scientific content of the British Pharmaceutical Conference (BPC); keeps the Council aware of scientific developments and UK science policy, and possible effects on pharmacy practice.
- **The Investigating Committee** is a key component of the fitness to practise committee structure. One of the functions of the Investigating Committee is to make initial decisions in relation to allegations of impairment of fitness to practise, by deciding whether to refer such allegations to other relevant parts of the committee structure.
- **The Adjudicating Committee** assesses pharmacists from outside the European Union (EU) who want to practise in the UK, and EU pharmacists who do not automatically qualify to register in the UK.
- **The Audit Committee** selects the Society's external and internal auditors, and reviews

the Society's financial control and risk-management systems, to ensure the reliability of its financial reporting.

- **The Conference Committee** is responsible for strategy, planning and development of the BPC. It is supported by the Programme Group, which develops the practice and science sessions of the BPC.
- **The Governance Committee** is responsible for ensuring that the Society operates in a legal and professional way, and meets commercial and financial requirements. It also advises the Council on how changes in legislation will affect the profession.
- **The Remuneration Committee** assesses remuneration for Society staff and agrees annual changes in remuneration for senior staff.

The National Pharmacy Boards

Until January 2007, the Society in Scotland and Wales was represented by the Scottish and Welsh Executives. The responsibilities of the Executives were to implement the policies of the Society, organisation and supervision of the local branches of the Society, and to make recommendations to the Council of matters affecting the Society and its members in Scotland and Wales (RPSGB, 2005).

Following political devolution in Great Britain, the Society formed the Devolution Review Group to conduct a review of its structure and function in England, Scotland and Wales. As a result of this review, it was proposed that the Scottish and Welsh Executives were replaced with national boards, and that an English board was created. The members of these boards were elected during 2006 and the boards were duly created on 21 January 2007. The boards are structured and function differently from each other, but the overall aim and purpose of them is the same; the remit of the boards is to:

1. provide strategic leadership and support for pharmacy practice development
2. assist development of Council policy and

its implementation, and develop and implement policy specific to each country
3. promote the science and practice of pharmacy and its contribution to health
4. provide professional advice to government and its agencies, National Health Services bodies, and other health and social care organisations
5. support the Society's branches in each country
6. support pharmacists in their professional roles.

Branches and regions of the RPSGB

The Council set up branches of the Society throughout Great Britain in 1922. Currently there are 136 local branches, with a membership comprising pharmacists resident in that area. Each branch elects a committee, which runs the branch and organises regular meetings, usually of an educational nature. Meetings often involve presentations by external speakers such as local hospital doctors and academic experts, who provide useful insights or updates on current therapeutic or research areas. Branch meetings are a good opportunity for networking with local pharmacists and a valuable source of CPD.

A regional organisation in England and Wales was set up in 1968. The regions supplement the branch structure and help smaller branches (Appelbe & Wingfield, 2005). They act as a link between the local branches and the Council, and are also involved in the coordination of public relations activities. The membership of regions is made up of the members of branches within each region.

The future of the RPSGB

The White Paper *Trust, assurance and safety – the regulation of health professionals in the 21st century* was published in February 2007 following a series of incidents involving harm to patients caused by doctors, most notably the Shipman case, and the findings of the inquiries into these incidents (Department of Health, 2007). This document sets out the Government's policy on regulation of all health professions, including pharmacy, and is likely to result in changes to the law pertaining to this.

The main recommendation relating to pharmacy will result in fundamental changes to the way the profession is regulated and represented. The White Paper recommends the formation of a General Pharmaceutical Council (GPhC) to take over the regulatory role of the RPSGB. It is likely that professional leadership will be taken over by a 'Royal College'-type organisation. These changes will bring the profession in line with other professions that are regulated and represented by different bodies. Examples include medicine: doctors must register with the General Medical Council in order to practise, and professional leadership is provided by a number of Royal Colleges, such as the Royal College of Physicians, the Royal College of Surgeons, the Royal College of Psychiatrists, etc. Similarly, nurses and midwives are regulated by the Nursing and Midwifery Council, and represented by the Royal College of Nursing (Department of Health, 2007).

This is an exciting time for the membership of the Society. It is an opportunity to look to the future of the profession and develop representative bodies that will be better suited to the role of regulation and representation of pharmacists and pharmacy technicians well into the 21st century.

Summary

The RPSGB has a long history stretching back well over 100 years. At the time of writing, however, the future of the Society is uncertain – it will survive, but it is not yet known in what form, and what the function will be. For the membership, it is an exciting time, as it is to be hoped that modernisation will produce a body fit to lead the profession for the next 100 years.

References

Appelbe G E, Wingfield J (2005) *Dale and Appelbe's Pharmacy Law and Ethics*. 8th edn. London: Pharmaceutical Press.

Department of Health (2007) *Trust, assurance and safety – the regulation of health professionals in the 21st century*. www.dh.gov.uk/en/Publicationsandstatistics/Publications/PublicationsPolicyAndGuidance/DH_065946

Homan P G (2002) Patent and brandname medicines. London: Museum of the Royal Pharmaceutical Society of Great Britain. www.rpsgb.org.uk/pdfs/mussheet10.pdf (accessed 10 September 2007)

RPSGB (2005) *Devolution – A Framework for the Future. The Fraser Report. Report of the RPSGB Devolution Review Group*. London: Royal Pharmaceutical Society of Great Britain.

RPSGB (2006). *Annual Review*. London: Royal Pharmaceutical Society of Great Britain.

Royal Charter of Incorporation (1843). London: Royal Pharmaceutical Society of Great Britain.

8

Essential communication skills for pharmacists

Kate E Fletcher

Introduction

Pharmacists must be able to communicate effectively with many different groups of people in order to carry out their job:

- patients and their carers
- other staff within the pharmacy
- nurses and doctors
- other health professionals such as physiotherapists and dietitians.

Pharmacists need to be able to communicate in various situations, and using different methods, whether it is face to face in the community pharmacy or hospital ward, over the telephone, making presentations at conferences, or writing letters and emails. The ability to tailor one's approach to communication in all its forms for all of these groups is therefore a critical skill that today's pharmacist has to develop. This chapter introduces some of the verbal and non-verbal skills required to communicate effectively in these settings.

Having good communication skills will also contribute to one of the most important attributes for a pharmacist, that is, professionalism (see Box 8.1). This is a difficult concept to define, but good communication skills contribute towards it.

Interacting with patients

The main skills required to interact successfully with patients are active listening, questioning, responding and explaining. Each of these skills is explained below.

Active listening

Listening is more than simply hearing a person speak to you. It should be an active process, ensuring not only that all messages are received but also that the speaker knows that the listener has understood the message. For pharmacists, this is particularly important when talking with patients. It is essential that the patient knows that the pharmacist is listening to them and taking their situation and opinions seriously. Patients – who may not be feeling well or may be shocked and/or concerned by a diagnosis, for

---

Box 8.1   Definitions of professionalism in pharmacy

Bumgarner *et al.* (2007) described professionalism as, 'the enactment of the values and ideals of individuals who are called, as pharmacists, to serve individuals and populations, whose care is entrusted to them, prioritising the interests of those they serve above their own . . .'

In an extensive review of professionalism in pharmacy, Hammer *et al.* (2003) conceptualised professionalism in pharmacy as a bicycle wheel. The centre consists of values associated with professionalism, such as altruism, caring, honour, integrity and duty. From this centre arise spokes, which represent behaviours associated with professionalism, such as respect, accountability, empathy and compassion. The outer tyre of the wheel represents the surface of professionalism, encompassing such things as professional attire, courtesy and punctuality.

Chisholm *et al.* (2006) listed the following ten broad traits that enable pharmacists and pharmacy students to act professionally:

- accountability for his/her actions
- commitment to self-improvement of skills and knowledge
- conscience and trustworthiness
- covenantal relationship with client (patient)
- creativity and innovation
- ethically sound decision making
- knowledge and skills of the profession
- leadership
- pride in the profession
- service oriented.

---

example – are easily intimidated by someone in a 'white coat'; by demonstrating good listening skills, the pharmacist can help the patient to feel much more comfortable and relaxed about their situation and the means by which it can be resolved. This in turn will help the pharmacist to obtain more useful information from the patient, as the patient will find it easier to share such information relating to themselves, enabling the pharmacist to fulfil their role more effectively. It is not unusual for a patient to give the pharmacist information that they may feel unable to share with their doctor or nurse, as many patients perceive pharmacists to be more understanding and approachable.

The three main techniques involved in active listening are:

- maintaining eye contact – so that the speaker can see you are paying attention
- acknowledging what the speaker says – by suitable body language such as nodding and verbal agreement
- summarising or paraphrasing what has just been said (e.g. using a phrase such 'So, what you're saying is. . .').

Questioning

Pharmacists need to use effective questioning in order to obtain information from patients, usually relating to their medication. It is important not to ask leading questions, as patients will sometimes just agree or go along with the lead, because they are afraid to get the question 'wrong'. For instance, when trying to identify which inhaler a patient uses when the patient doesn't know the name of the inhaler, the pharmacist might want to find out what colour it is, as different types have a specific colour. A leading question would be, 'Is your inhaler blue?' However, the patient may be tempted to reply 'yes' to this as it might appear to be the 'right' answer. A better way to ask is, 'What colour is your inhaler?' Without giving the patient a colour, they are not prompted, and will hopefully remember what colour the inhaler actually is. This type of questioning also makes it is easier and more likely for a patient to admit that they don't know the answer.

Getting accurate information with regard to a medication history is essential, as this will result in the patient receiving the correct medication while they are in hospital. In this example, if the information regarding the patient's inhalers is not correct, the wrong medications might be prescribed, resulting in a loss of control of the patient's asthma, and therefore the potential for a life-threatening asthma attack to occur.

There are three main types of questioning.

- **Open questions** have no right or wrong answer and there is usually more than one possible answer, for example, 'Please describe . . .?' or 'Tell me about. . .?' Open questions are used to obtain general information. An open question may be followed by a closed or probing question based on part of the answer, to obtain more precise or detailed information.
- **Closed or convergent questions** home in or converge on specific information. Examples are questions that have a right or wrong answer such as, 'What is your name?' or questions that are answered with yes or no: 'Are you John Smith?'
- **Probing questions** are used to obtain specific information. They may be used to clarify previous answers, or to elaborate on information obtained by open questioning. For example: 'Please tell me about the medication you take' might be followed by, 'What is the name of the tablet you take for your high blood pressure?'

Responding and explaining

Using active listening techniques (see above) will help demonstrate respect, understanding and empathy with the patient. This in turn will help you earn the trust and respect of the patient, and build an effective professional relationship with them, enabling you to do your job as a pharmacist more effectively. It also is important to be confident when talking with patients, so they have confidence in what you tell them. It is unlikely that a patient will trust a health professional who is hesitant or doesn't appear confident about what they are talking about.

When explaining something to a patient, such as how to use an inhaler, it is essential to use language and concepts that the patient will understand. Technical words and jargon should never be used, as many patients will not understand such terms, and they might not have the confidence to ask for a further explanation. The level at which information can be pitched varies between individuals, and with experience it is possible to assess how well a patient understands the information you have given them.

It is often necessary to check that a patient understands information you have given them, but in doing so it is important not to patronise them. A good method of checking understanding is to ask the patient to explain something back to you, for instance, after explaining how to use an inhaler, ask the patient to explain it back to you.

Interacting with other health professionals

Talking with other health professionals is very different from talking with patients. This can be quite intimidating for the pre-registration or newly qualified pharmacist, especially when talking to doctors, as they might ask questions or require explanations that the pharmacist may not be prepared for. This may be because of lack of experience or specialist knowledge of the clinical speciality in question, and becomes less

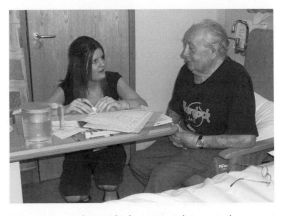

Figure 8.1   A hospital pharmacist discusses drug treatment with a patient. Her position enables her to speak easily with the patient.

common as a pharmacist becomes more experienced. The principal key, therefore, to successful interactions with doctors and other health professionals is preparation.

If you need to get information from other people, think about what you want to know, and then the questions you need to ask to get that information. If necessary, write the questions down, so you don't forget any of them, and then arrange your questions in a logical order. Having to go back to a person repeatedly because you've forgotten something is embarrassing and is likely to annoy them!

If you are talking to a prescriber about a change in treatment, make sure you can justify your suggestion with evidence, and can also supply prescribing information for the alternative choice of treatment, thereby proffering a solution to the issue rather than barriers to successful treatment of the patient.

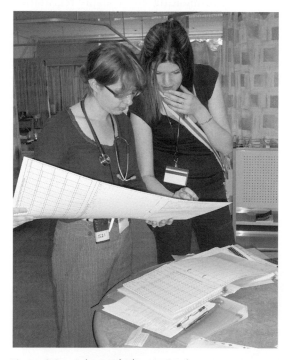

Figure 8.2 A hospital pharmacist discusses a patient's drug treatment with a junior doctor.

Presentations

Presentations are an important part of many pharmacy undergraduate programmes, and continue to be part of the role of the qualified pharmacist, particularly in primary care and hospital settings. This section discusses how to plan a presentation, decide on content, design slides and use appropriate body language and voice skills to make a good presentation (Box 8.2).

Planning the presentation

The first steps in planning a presentation are to know how long the presentation should be, and to establish the aim of the presentation. Is it to inform the audience, to educate them, or to persuade and change opinions or attitudes? Once you have determined the purpose, it is easier to decide on the appropriate content, structure and style of the presentation.

Next think about the topic(s) you want to cover, and then arrange them in a logical order so that each slide leads on to the next. This will help your audience to follow you more easily. It is a good idea to start with an outline or overview of the presentation, so the audience immediately knows what you are going to talk about. Let them know how long you will be talking for and when they can ask questions (i.e. during or after the presentation).

End your presentation with a summary and conclusion. This allows you to reiterate and reinforce the main points of the presentation. It also enables you to create a lasting positive impression, as the last things you say will be those most easily remembered by the audience.

Make sure you prepare for possible questions you might be asked. One way to do this is to ask a colleague to listen to your presentation and to tell you what questions they would ask; prepare answers for these.

In order to pitch the content at the right level, think about who your audience is. Pharmacists may be required to present to nurses, doctors and other pharmacists. These different groups will be interested in different parts of the same subject. For instance, if a hospital pharmacist is giving a presentation on a new drug, doctors will be most interested in indications for use, how to prescribe it and monitoring parameters. Nurses will want to know how to give it safely and how to monitor the patient immediately after it is given. Pharmacists will want to know all of these things, and more!

Preparing slides

Most people now use computers to design and project their slides. However, it is worth considering making a 'hard' copy on overhead projector (OHP) slides, in case your disk or memory stick corrupts, or the projection equipment fails or is not available.

Slides should:

- be simple and uncluttered
- have a balanced even layout
- show content in a way that is easily assimilated – it is often better to use several short slides than one complex one
- be easy to present.

Some examples of bad and good slides are shown in Figures 8.3 and 8.4.

Abbreviations, acronyms and technical terms should be defined on the first use, to ensure all members of the audience understand them. Animation should only be used if it enhances your presentation. Excessive animation can be distracting and detract from the content of the presentation.

If you use OHP slides, if possible they should be printed or photocopied. In use, make sure they are correctly orientated on the OHP, and that the OHP is in focus. Try not to fiddle with them, as this is distracting for the audience and makes them more difficult to read. You may want to cover part of the slide and reveal it later, so that the audience doesn't get ahead of you.

Using notes or cue cards

Some people like to use some form of notes to help them remember the content of their presentation. These can take the form of cue cards with bullet points, or a longhand version on paper. It

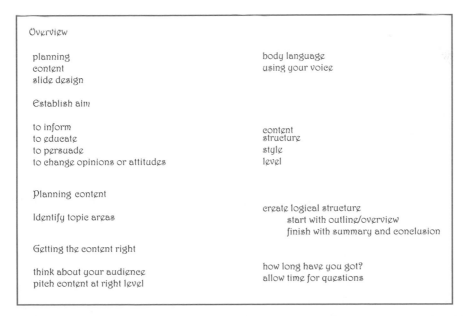

Figure 8.3   A poorly prepared slide: the font is small and difficult to read, the information is cramped, and there is too much information on the slide.

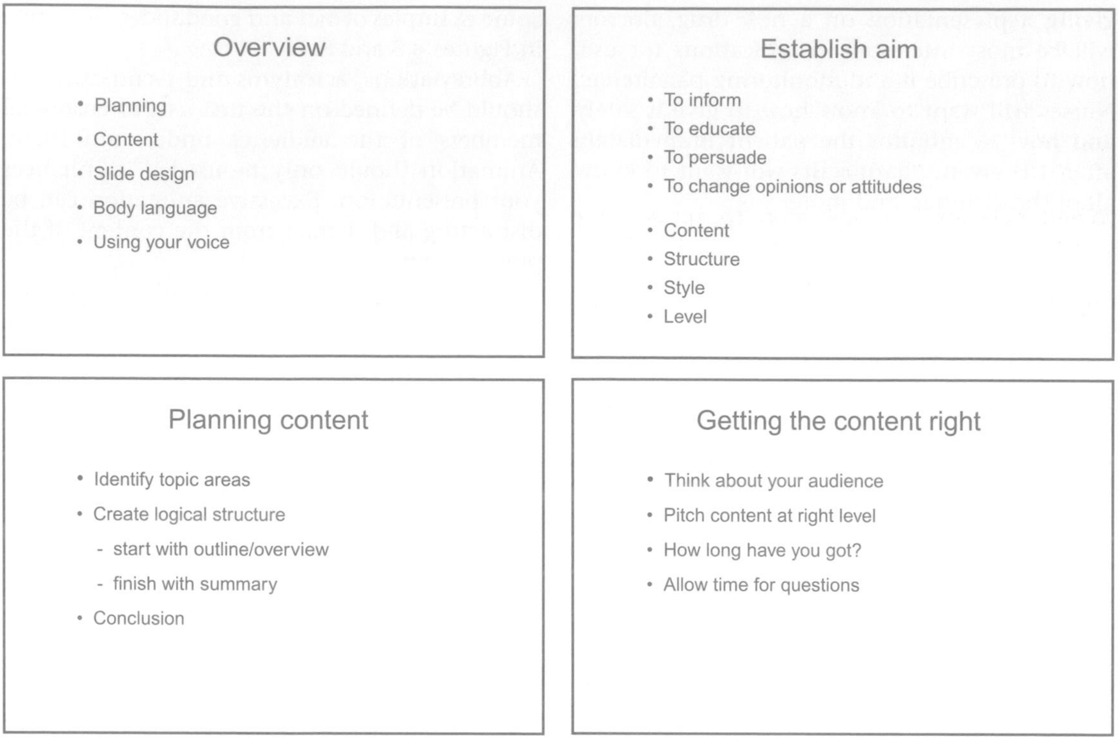

Overview	Establish aim
• Planning • Content • Slide design • Body language • Using your voice	• To inform • To educate • To persuade • To change opinions or attitudes • Content • Structure • Style • Level

Planning content	Getting the content right

• Identify topic areas
• Create logical structure
   - start with outline/overview
   - finish with summary
• Conclusion
	• Think about your audience
	• Pitch content at right level
	• How long have you got?
	• Allow time for questions

Figure 8.4   Some examples of well prepared slides. The font is large and clear; the information is laid out clearly with bullet points; there is not too much information on each slide.

is important not to use these too much, as this will affect your presentation style; you will not be able to make eye contact and are less likely to come across as being confident and knowledgeable if you are reading from notes. It is a good idea to practise your talk several times, especially if you are not used to giving presentations, in order to reduce reliance on prompts. Use the words on the slides as prompts to help you remember what to say.

Using your voice

The voice is the main instrument of communication, so it is important you use it effectively when giving a presentation. The voice is vulnerable to stress, so before and during the presentation, try to stay relaxed; breathe deeply and keep your shoulders and arms relaxed. Have a glass of water handy in case your throat gets dry.

The voice can be adversely affected by laryngeal irritants, so it is best to avoid certain things before giving a presentation. These include smoking, spirits (they may feel soothing but in fact they anaesthetise the throat while causing further irritation), smoky, dusty and dry atmospheres, coffee and tea, hot spicy food, gargling, indigestion and heartburn (Mathieson, 2007).

Speak clearly and distinctly so that your audience can hear you. Open your mouth well when speaking, to avoid mumbling. If possible, go to the room you are presenting in before the day, so you know how big it is. Practise speaking in it with a friend listening in different parts of the room to check your volume is right.

It might be useful to try some voice exercises to warm up your voice and help you speak clearly. For example, try these phrases, which need to be enunciated carefully to be easy to hear and understand (Van Emden & Becker, 2004):

- electromagnetic compatibility (is every 't' clear?)
- romantics, realists and impressionists (avoid saying 'dimpressionists')
- peas, beans, broccoli and cauliflowers (makes your mouth work hard).

When nervous it is common to speak more quickly than usual, which can make it difficult for people to hear everything you say, so try to slow down. Nervousness can also make you speak in a higher pitch than usual, so be aware of this and use a pitch that is comfortable for you to avoid straining your voice. Ensure that you complete each sentence clearly. It is common for the voice to tail off towards the end of a sentence.

Make sure you address everyone. Appropriate body language will help your voice skills (see below).

Practising your presentation a few times before giving it will help you improve your presentation style, and, if you are nervous, will give you more confidence, as you will be more familiar with the content.

Most importantly, be yourself! If you have a strong accent, don't try to change it, but it may be particularly important to speak slowly and clearly, so the audience can hear and understand you.

Body language

Using the right body language will help you make a more effective presentation. Think about the people who have given presentations to you. The good ones usually use friendly open body language, and engage with their audience; bad speakers may not make eye contact, and turn towards the screen rather than face the audience and engage with them.

When giving a presentation, try to have good eye contact with the audience as a whole; don't just stare at one person, you'll make them feel uncomfortable! Adopt a relaxed posture, with your head up and level; this will enhance your voice and make you easier to hear. Face the audience and make open arm gestures. Don't fold

---

Box 8.2   Giving a presentation

1. Plan the content
   Consider:
   - aim
   - length
   - audience
   Include:
   - overview
   - summary.
2. Designing slides
   Slides should be:
   - simple
   - clear
   - easy to understand
   - easy to present
3. Using notes or cue cards
   - do not use as script

4. Using your voice
   - practice
   - speak slowly and clearly
   - stay relaxed
   - breathe deeply
   - have drinking water handy
5. Body language
   - relax
   - open posture
   - eye contact
   - smile!
6. Room layout and equipment
   - Arrive early
   - rearrange if necessary
   - check equipment works
   - check your presentation works on the computer set-up provided

your arms, this will come across as unfriendly, and the audience will be less likely to engage with you. And don't forget to smile!

Room layout and equipment

If possible, go to the room in which you will be presenting before the day, so you can see how the room is laid out. You might want to change the layout for your presentation, so on the day get there early so you have time to move things around. Familiarise yourself with the computer and projection equipment, and make sure it all works. Doing this early can prevent any embarrassing mishaps after your audience has arrived.

Summary

This chapter demonstrates how effective communication involves much more than merely talking to people. The pharmacy student must master various forms of communication such as presentation skills, active listening, open, closed and probing questioning, and be aware of how body language can be used to aid communication. By learning about and using these techniques, you will become a more confident and effective pharmacist.

References

Bumgarner G W, Spies A R, Asbill C S, Prince V T (2007). Using the humanities to strengthen the concept of professionalism among first-professional year pharmacy students. *Am J Pharm Educ* 71: 28.

Chisholm M A, Cobb H, Duke L, *et al.* (2006). Development of an instrument to measure professionalism. *Am J Pharm Educ* 70: 85.

Hammer D P, Berger B A, Beardsley R S, Easton M R (2003). Student professionalism. *Am J Pharm Educ* 67: 96.

Mathieson L (2007). *Personal communication*. London: University College London.

Useful resources

Goodlad S (1996). *Speaking technically. a handbook for scientists, engineers, and physicians on how to improve technical presentations*. London: Imperial College Press.

Van Emden J, Becker L (2004). *Presentation skills for students*. Basingstoke: Palgrave Macmillan.

9

Prescriptions – types and legal requirements

Sam E Weston

Introduction

This chapter describes current prescription forms seen in primary care. These forms are often updated, but they provide examples of the types of prescription form you might see during your career.

Types of medicine

At the time of writing, the Medicines Act (1968) classifies medicines into three categories:

- general sales list (GSL)
- pharmacy medicine (P)
- prescription only medicine (POM).

GSL medicines are available to the public through many outlets, from supermarkets to the local garage. These are medicines which have a history of being safe and effective, meaning they can be sold by a person with no medical or pharmacy training.

'P' medicines are available only from pharmacies and can only be sold under the supervision of a pharmacist. Some 'P' medicines are products that have been deregulated from POM status, whereas others may have potential for misuse or require the supervision of a pharmacist during the sale. Other 'P' medicines need a pharmacist's expert knowledge of drug actions and possible interactions in order to be supplied to patients in certain situations. For example, a patient who is taking certain antihypertensives should not take the decongestants that are included in many cold and flu remedies, as the two drugs can interact and cause an increase in the patient's blood pressure. Another example is the use of antihistamines for hay fever symptoms: people who use machinery or drive as part of their daily life should be counter-prescribed a non-drowsy once-a-day antihistamine.

POMs are only available on a prescription from an authorised prescriber (as currently defined by the Medicines Act 1968). The prescription may be either on a National Health Service (NHS) prescription form (subsidised) by the government, or a private prescription, the full cost of which is to be paid for by the patient. Authorised prescribers include a variety of health professionals such as general practitioners (GPs), dentists, podiatrists, pharmacists, health visitors, physiotherapists, chiropodists, practice nurses, optometrists, hospital doctors and radiographers, and also veterinary surgeons. Although these health professionals can all prescribe medications, all have some form of restriction placed on them as to the range of medication they can prescribe. GPs can prescribe any medication at NHS expense except those listed in Part XVIIIA of the *Drug Tariff* (published monthly and available online at www.drugtariff.com to registered users). This section of the *Drug Tariff* contains information on medicines and other substances that cannot be prescribed under the NHS Pharmaceutical Services, sometimes known as the 'black list' (a list of drugs that have been deemed as unsuitable for prescription on the NHS on the grounds of efficacy, cost or other issues). In addition, prescribers are advised to adhere to local formulary guidelines, agreed between the Department of Health, local primary care trusts and hospital trusts in that region. Dentists can prescribe items listed in the *Dental Practitioner Formulary* (DPF) and nurses from the *Nurse Practitioner Formulary*. (Both can be found in the back of the *British National Formulary* (BNF).) However, it is important to note that doctors and dentists can prescribe any POM on a private prescription, and are not confined to formulary guidelines that apply when prescribing on an NHS prescription form. This is discussed in more detail below, in the section on private prescriptions (page 91). Note also that unlicensed medications can be prescribed by qualified doctors under certain circumstances – such as when no other suitable medication is available to treat a patient with a certain illness. These unlicensed medications are not listed in the *Drug Tariff*, so pharmacists need to be aware of information sources that are available for such products (e.g. BNF), in the event that a prescription is presented to them for dispensing.

Prescribers

Historically, only doctors were allowed to prescribe. However, the first *Crown Report* published in 1998 recommended changes to the prescribing system and, as a result, nurse prescribing was piloted and then introduced throughout England from 1998, with a successful outcome. Since publication of the second *Crown Report* in 1999, pharmacists have also joined the ranks of prescribers – both as independent prescribers and supplementary prescribers (originally known as dependent prescribers).

- Independent prescribers assess patients, make diagnoses and prescribe suitable medication – this is linked to the role of community pharmacists within their extended role as prescribers in minor ailment schemes (see Chapter 3).
- Supplementary prescribers are responsible for maintaining the continuation of care of a patient previously diagnosed by a physician; this encompasses the role of pharmacists in the maintenance of patient care in hospital settings (see Chapter 4).

Prescription forms

Prescription forms are currently paper documents, which may be handwritten, typed or computer generated. The prescription gives details of the medicine(s) to be dispensed for a named patient and is issued by an authorised prescriber, as detailed above. The medication can be from any of the categories listed at the start of the chapter.

A prescription item is a single named medication on a prescription (e.g. aspirin 75 mg dispersible tablets). However, a prescription may contain more than one prescription item (e.g. aspirin 75 mg dispersible tablets and paracetamol 500 mg tablets), making the prescription form a multiple-item prescription. Prescriptions do not necessarily include only medications; items such as wound dressings, gluten-free food products, stoma appliances and elastic hosiery may be included on a prescription form.

Electronic prescriptions are the latest development in NHS prescription forms. Since the publication of the NHS Plan in 2000

(Department of Health, 2000), there has been a steady move towards the routine use of electronic prescriptions in both community and hospital environments. Electronic prescriptions will have the same legal force as a paper prescription and will eventually replace the latter completely. The benefits of electronic prescriptions include

- patient convenience
- easier ordering of repeat prescriptions
- availability of more complete information about prescribing to all members of a healthcare team.

By transferring information about the prescriber's choice of medication for a patient electronically, a more holistic picture about the treatment regimen can be seen by any member of the healthcare team, which will, in turn, improve the continuity of the patient's care. The only exception to the transformation from paper to electronic format will be private prescriptions, which will remain paper based for the immediate future.

Information required on a prescription

A prescription is a means of communication between the prescriber and the pharmacist. The minimum information and instructions that are required are shown in Box 9.1.

Types of prescription form

NHS prescriptions

Prescription forms currently exist in many guises. Prescription forms must be used for prescribing POMs and appliances. In addition, each prescribing group (doctors, dentists, nurses, etc.) is restricted in the prescription form that they can use. The information below was correct at the time of writing (December 2007). Up-to-date information can be obtained via the Prescription Pricing Division website: www.ppa.org.uk.

Box 9.1   Essential information to be included on a National Health Service prescription form

- **Name, address and telephone number of the prescriber** – this allows the prescriber to be contacted in the event of any problems with interpreting the prescription.
- **Date of the prescription** – some legislation governing dispensing requires certain medicines to be dispensed within a certain time from the date on the prescription (e.g. controlled drugs).
- **Name of the medicine, strength and dosage form** – in the UK it is advised that medicines are written using their generic (or approved) name (i.e. the name of the drug) rather than their proprietary or brand name. This is also sometimes referred to as the recommended international non-proprietary name (rINN). However, the brand name can be written for exceptions where it important that a patient receives the same dosage form; this is particularly the case with many drugs used to treat epilepsy.

- **Dose and dosing regimen** – this allows the pharmacist to ensure that the correct dose has been prescribed for the patient; note, however, that some products (e.g. creams and ointments), may not have a specific dose.
- **Total amount to be dispensed** – this can be written as a quantity or as the length of treatment course, for example 21 capsules can be written as '21' or as 'one capsule, three times a day for 7 days'.
- **Directions for use** – this includes instruction on how a medicinal product should be used (e.g. 'spread thinly' in the case of steroid creams).
- **Name and address** of the patient (and age if under 12 years old).
- **Prescriber's signature** – this must be in indelible ink.

Prescription forms used in England

Prescription forms currently used in England are carefully divided to ensure that each prescriber uses the correct type of form. Table 9.1 lists the majority of prescription forms used in England at the time of writing, their unique identifying codes, colours describing differences between them, who uses each form type and for what purpose. The potential for fraudulent reproduction and abuse of the prescribing system is of obvious concern to health professionals and the authorities; because of this, all NHS prescription forms are now made of special paper that makes them virtually impossible to scan, photocopy or reproduce in any way, in order to minimise this risk. For this reason we cannot show images of the range of prescription forms, although an image of a blank English FP10 has been used in Chapter 10 to identify different sections of the prescription form for interpretation by the pharmacist.

Prescription forms used in Wales

From March 2004, Welsh prescribers began using new bilingual prescription forms with the identifier code 'WP10'. Both English and Welsh language text appear on the forms. These forms can be presented for dispensing at pharmacies in England, and should be dispensed from in the usual manner. All WP10 forms are green but are easily identifiable by the presence of The Welsh Assembly Government (dragon) logo in the bottom-left corner and the NHS Wales logo in the bottom-right corner.

Each individual prescriber group or type of prescription is further identifiable by the code printed at the bottom of the prescription (e.g. dentists prescribe on WP10D followed by the individual form serial number). In addition, the prescriber type is printed alongside the 'Date of Birth' and under the 'Name' box. The paper and security measures incorporated in the prescription form are the same as the current English

Table 9.1 Prescription forms used in England

Paper type	Colour	Type of form	For use by	Patients
FP10NC	Green	Preprinted green form for computer-generated prescriptions	GPs Hospital-based prescribers	Practice patients Outpatient clinics
FP10SS	Green	Blank green form for computer-generated or handwritten prescriptions	GPs (and hospitals or supplementary prescribers using accredited systems)	Practice patients Outpatient clinics
FP10MDA	Blue	Drug misuse instalment prescriptions, can be preprinted or blank forms	GPs Hospital-based prescribers Supplementary prescribers	Registered addicts
FP10P	Lilac	Handwritten prescriptions	For use by nurses, supplementary or additional prescribers and out-of-hours centres	Home visit patients Patients visiting a nurse-led clinic Emergency patients
FP10D	Yellow	Blank yellow form for computer-generated or handwritten prescriptions	Community dentist	Practice patients Emergency patients
FP10PCDSS	Pink	Computer-generated or handwritten single-sheet prescription for controlled drugs	GPs	Practice patients Home visit patients Emergency patients

Adapted from information presented on the Prescriptions Pricing Authority website (www.ppa.org.uk)

Table 9.2   Prescription forms used in Wales

Paper type	Colour	Purpose	For use by	Patients
WP10NC	Green	Preprinted green form for computer-generated prescriptions	GPs Hospital-based prescribers	Practice patients Outpatient clinics
WP10SS	Green	Blank green form for computer-generated or handwritten prescriptions	GPs (and hospitals or supplementary prescribers using accredited systems)	Practice patients Outpatient clinics
WP10MDA	Green Blue	Drug misuse instalment prescriptions, can be preprinted or blank forms	GPs Hospital-based prescribers Supplementary prescribers	Registered addicts
WP10HP	Green Orange		Hospital based prescribers	Outpatient clinics
WP10CN	Green Purple	Handwritten or computer-generated prescriptions	Community nurses	Home visit patients Patients visiting a nurse-led clinic Emergency patients
WP10PN	Green Purple	Handwritten or computer-generated prescriptions	Practice nurses	Home visit patients Patients visiting a nurse-led clinic Emergency patients
WP10D	Green Yellow		Community dentist	Practice patients Emergency patients
WP10SP	Green		Supplementary prescribers	Patients who do not need referral to a GP

Adapted from National Pharmacy Association *Drug Tariff Handbook*

FP10 series. Table 9.2 outlines the major prescription forms used in Wales.

Prescription forms used in Scotland

Scottish prescriptions also differ slightly from the prescription forms seen in England, and a specific category of prescription exists solely for use by pharmacists. The categories of prescriber allowed to prescribe on each form type are also different. Table 9.3 outlines the major prescription forms used in Scotland.

Prescription forms used in Northern Ireland

In Northern Ireland, prescription forms are currently divided into four categories. There are currently no specific forms for use by pharmacists, but local health authority schemes are in place to allow prescribing by accredited pharmacists for minor ailment scheme. Table 9.4 outlines the major prescription forms used in Northern Ireland.

Other prescription forms in use

The Isle of Man, Jersey and Guernsey have separate prescriptions. The prescription forms specific for Jersey and Guernsey can only be filled in on the island on which they are issued. Recently, prescription forms specifically used for the supply of Schedules 2 and 3 controlled drugs (FP10PCD) by a prescriber have been introduced for patients collecting medications from a community pharmacy. These are still relatively uncommon, as their introduction is being

Table 9.3   Prescription forms used in Scotland

Paper type	Colour	Purpose	For use by	Patients
GP10/GP10SS	Orange	Preprinted green form for computer-generated prescriptions	GPs Hospital-based prescribers	Practice patients Outpatient clinics
GP10A	Pink	Ordering stock items for practice or medical bags No equivalent in England or Wales	GPs	
GP10DTS	Pink		Drug testing scheme officers	Registered addicts
GP10(N)	Purple		Nurse prescribers, including independent and supplementary prescribers	General practice patients
GP14	Yellow		Community dentist	Practice patients Emergency patients
CP2	Yellow		Pharmacists	Patients with minor ailments
CPUS	Yellow	Urgent supply of medication to a patient	Pharmacists	
HBP	Blue		Hospital-based prescribers	Outpatient supply
HBP(A)	Pink		Hospital clinics – for supply of medication to registered drug addicts	

Adapted from National Pharmacy Association *Drug Tariff Handbook*

Table 9.4   Prescription forms used in Northern Ireland

Paper type	Colour	Purpose	For use by	Patients
HS21	Green	Preprinted green form for computer-generated prescriptions	GPs Hospital-based prescribers	Practice patients Outpatient clinics
HS21S	White	Ordering stock items for practice or medical bags No equivalent in England or Wales	GPs	
HS21D	Yellow		Community dentist	Practice patients Emergency patients
HS21N	Purple		Nurse prescribers, including independent and supplementary prescribers	General practice patients

Adapted from National Pharmacy Association *Drug Tariff Handbook*

phased in as old-style prescription forms are used up. Both the old- and the new-style prescription forms have a space on the back for the signature of the person collecting the medication. In the longer term, further changes will be made to allocate each prescriber with a unique code to allow more accurate monitoring of the prescribing of controlled drugs.

Private prescriptions

Currently POM, 'P' and GSL category medicines can be supplied from a pharmacy when the pharmacist is presented with a private prescription. Although prescribers are governed by the *Drug Tariff* and various national formularies when prescribing on an FP10, WP10, GP10 or HS21 form, prescribers are allowed to order any POM, 'P' or GSL medicine on a private prescription form (RPSGB, 2007).

Details that must be included on a private prescription in order for it to be valid include:

- a signature and the prescriber's name in indelible ink
- the address of practitioner supplying the prescription
- an appropriate date
- the qualification details of prescriber
- name and address of the patient (and age if less than 12 years old).

In order to confirm the registration details of a prescribing doctor or dentist, pharmacists have access to the General Medical Council list of registered medical practitioners and the General Dental Council register online to check that the presciber is legally registered and therefore allowed to prescribe medications.

Hospital prescription forms

There is no standard prescription form used for hospital prescribing for inpatients, and the format varies from one hospital trust to another. (In reality, the chart used to record inpatient medication is known as 'an authority to administer'.) However, all forms have space for prescription details, as well as space for confirming that the medicine has been administered to the patient by a member of nursing or medical staff. Generally, hospital prescriptions are divided into four or five sections: regularly administered medicines; once-only medication; intermittent injections; continuous infusions; there may also be separate sections for the administration of blood products or drugs with variable doses, such as warfarin. Finally, the majority of hospital prescription forms include a section for 'as required' medication, which includes medicines such as analgesics (painkillers), laxatives, etc., that can be given to the patient by nursing staff at their discretion, without the need for a doctor to add the medication to the regular medications section of the prescription form. These items can be written up before they are needed, together with directions for maximum daily dose and dosing interval for the nursing staff to use in the event the patient requires the medication. Figure 9.1 is an example of a hospital prescription form used for teaching undergraduate students.

Veterinary prescriptions

In 2002 the Competition Commission published a report on veterinary medicines which outlined a monopoly situation in which veterinarians were prescribing and supplying medicines to pet owners. Recommendations have therefore been made to encourage the supply of veterinary medications from pharmacies, and pharmacists are increasingly being presented with veterinary prescriptions.

A 'veterinary medicinal product' can be supplied in accordance with a prescription. There are no standard forms, so most veterinary prescriptions take the form of a private prescription. In addition to the details included on a private prescription, a veterinary prescription must also contain:

- the name and address of the owner or keeper of the animal(s)
- the species of animal, identification and number of animal(s)
- the premises at which the animal(s) is/are kept if different from that of the owner or keeper.

The pharmacist should ensure that the prescriber is legally registered and entitled to prescribe the medication on the prescription.

Signed orders

A signed order can be accepted by a pharmacist for the supply of a Schedule 1 poison to a person

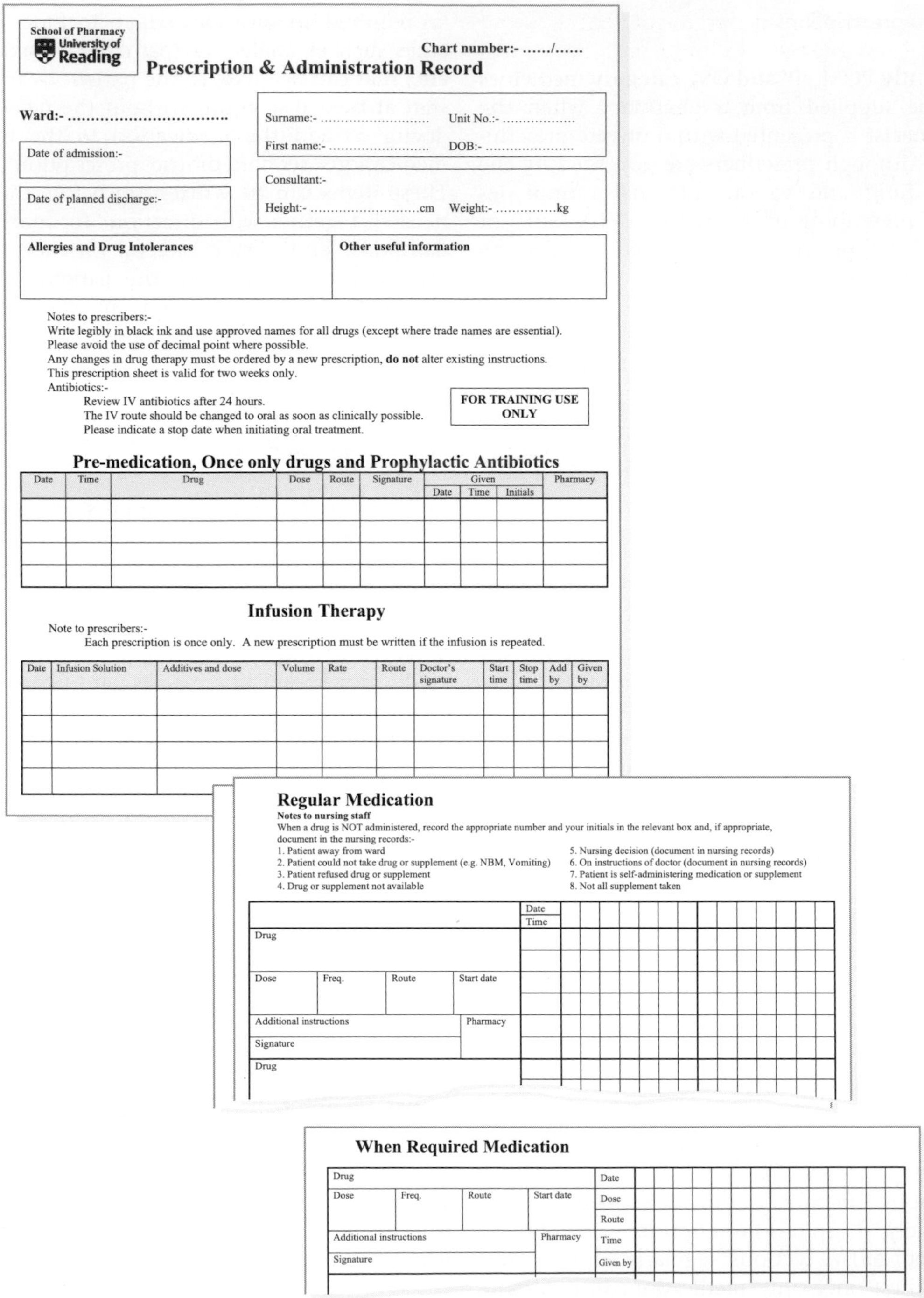

School of Pharmacy
University of Reading

Chart number:- ....../......

Prescription & Administration Record

Ward:- ....

Surname:- .... Unit No.:- ....

First name:- .... DOB:- ....

Date of admission:-

Consultant:-

Date of planned discharge:-

Height:- ....cm Weight:- ....kg

Allergies and Drug Intolerances	Other useful information

Notes to prescribers:-
Write legibly in black ink and use approved names for all drugs (except where trade names are essential).
Please avoid the use of decimal point where possible.
Any changes in drug therapy must be ordered by a new prescription, **do not** alter existing instructions.
This prescription sheet is valid for two weeks only.
Antibiotics:-
Review IV antibiotics after 24 hours.
The IV route should be changed to oral as soon as clinically possible.
Please indicate a stop date when initiating oral treatment.

FOR TRAINING USE ONLY

Pre-medication, Once only drugs and Prophylactic Antibiotics

Date	Time	Drug	Dose	Route	Signature	Given			Pharmacy
						Date	Time	Initials	

Infusion Therapy

Note to prescribers:-
Each prescription is once only. A new prescription must be written if the infusion is repeated.

Date	Infusion Solution	Additives and dose	Volume	Rate	Route	Doctor's signature	Start time	Stop time	Add by	Given by

Regular Medication

Notes to nursing staff
When a drug is NOT administered, record the appropriate number and your initials in the relevant box and, if appropriate, document in the nursing records:-
1. Patient away from ward
2. Patient could not take drug or supplement (e.g. NBM, Vomiting)
3. Patient refused drug or supplement
4. Drug or supplement not available
5. Nursing decision (document in nursing records)
6. On instructions of doctor (document in nursing records)
7. Patient is self-administering medication or supplement
8. Not all supplement taken

Date
Time
Drug
Dose | Freq. | Route | Start date
Additional instructions | Pharmacy
Signature
Drug

When Required Medication

Drug | Date
Dose | Freq. | Route | Start date | Dose
Route
Additional instructions | Pharmacy | Time
Signature | Given by

Figure 9.1 A hospital prescription chart currently used as an undergraduate teaching resource at the University of Reading, School of Pharmacy (modified from a prescription chart used at Oxford Radcliffe Hospitals NHS Trust). It consists of four pages: the first page gives the patient details, premedication, once-only drugs and prophylactic antibiotics, and infusion therapy; the second and third pages list regular medications; page 4 lists medications that can be administered as required.

who requires it for the purpose of their trade; for example, a pest control officer may require strychnine or fluoroacetic acid to be used as a poison for moles or rodents. In this situation, the 'prescription' or signed order must include:

- a signature in indelible ink
- the name and address of the purchaser
- details of their trade or profession
- the total quantity to be purchased
- the purpose for which the poison is required.

In addition to poisons, the community pharmacist may see signed orders for medicines and dressings for an on-call doctor's bag or for supplies for clinics held within a GP surgery. In a hospital environment, pharmacists will often receive signed orders from ward staff, and particularly from operating theatre staff, for the supply of controlled drugs for stock purposes. This ensures that a supply of medication is available in an emergency situation or when the pharmacy is closed.

Exemptions

Some exemptions apply to GSL, 'P' medicines and POMs. Certain groups of people are allowed to have these medicines supplied without the use of a prescription. These groups include:

- hospitals and health centres
- practitioners – doctors and dentists
- appropriate nurse prescribers
- midwives
- chiropodists
- optometrists
- drug treatment services
- owners and masters of ships
- operator or commander of an aircraft
- Royal National Lifeboat Institution
- British Red Cross Society
- occupational health schemes
- first aid personnel on offshore installations (such as oil rigs)
- ambulance paramedics
- universities.

Up-to-date details of the restrictions and regulations surrounding these and other groups are given in the *Medicines, Ethics and Practice Guide*

for Pharmacists and Pharmacy Technicians. An order can be provided by the purchaser in addition to details of their exemption status. It is good practice to record details of any sale or supply of POMs to any of the exempted groups of people described above in the prescription-only register. Details to be recorded include:

- the date on which the POM was sold or supplied
- the name, quantity, pharmaceutical form and strength of the medicine
- the name, address, trade, business or profession of the person to whom the medicine has been sold or supplied
- the purpose for which it was sold or supplied.

Restriction to medicines and appliances prescribed on NHS FP10 (and variations) forms

Schedule 1 products and appliances

Schedule 1 to the *NHS (General Medical Services Contract) (Prescription of Drugs) Regulations 2004* lists medicinal product and appliances that cannot be prescribed under NHS pharmaceutical services. This list is in Part XVIIIA of the *Drug Tariff* and is commonly known as the 'black list'. The Prescription Pricing Division (PPD) will not reimburse the dispensing contractor for items dispensed from this list.

Schedule 2 products and appliances

Schedule 2 to the *NHS (General Medical Services Contract) (Prescription of Drugs) Regulations 2004* lists drugs that may be prescribed in certain circumstances. The groups of patients who may receive these drugs for specific purposes are listed, but these drugs may not be prescribed to other types of patient or for different purposes. This list of drugs is called the 'selected list' and is found in Part XVIIIB of the *Drug Tariff*. The prescriber must endorse the FP10 with the term 'SLS' (selected list scheme) for the prescription to be accepted for processing by the PPD.

For example, cyanocobalamin tablets may be prescribed for the treatment or prevention of vitamin B12 deficiency in patients who are vegan or have a proven vitamin B12 deficiency of dietary origin. Appliances listed in Part IX of the *Drug Tariff* may be supplied on FP10.

Borderline substances

'Borderline substances include certain foods and toilet preparations. These products are divided into List A and List B and can be found in Part XV of the *Drug Tariff*. The prescriber must endorse the prescription specifically with the term 'ACBS'. The Advisory Committee on Borderline Substances (ACBS) advises when preparations may be regarded as drugs. An example is HCU gel, a methionine-free protein substitute for use in the dietary management of homocystinuria in children between the ages of 12 months and 10 years.

Non-GP prescribers

Dentists

Dentists are restricted to a specific list of products that can be prescribed on FP10D and should use the DPF. The PPD will only reimburse the dispensing contractor if the products are in the DPF. The most up-to-date list of preparations suitable for prescribing on FP10D are listed in Part XVIIA of the *Drug Tariff*. Note that private dental prescriptions are not restricted to the DPF.

Nurse prescribers

Two formularies exist for independent nurse prescribers:

- District nurse and health visitor prescribers can only prescribe preparations in Part XVIIB(i) of the *Drug Tariff*.
- Independent nurse prescribers (previously known as extended formulary nurse prescribers) can prescribe the above, plus

the list of products in Part XVIIB(ii) of the *Drug Tariff*. This specific section of the *Drug Tariff* is the most up-to-date record of products available in the nurse prescribers' formularies.

Supplementary prescribers

Supplementary prescribers can prescribe (provided they are included within the patient-specific clinical management plan):

- all GSL medicines, 'P' medicines, appliances and devices, foods and other borderline substances
- all POMs
- controlled drugs (Schedule 1 drugs not intended for medicinal use, e.g. poisons)
- medicines for use outside their licensed indications
- unlicensed drugs.

References

Competition Commission (2002). *Veterinary Medicines: A report on the supply within the United Kingdom of prescription-only veterinary medicines Volumes 1 & 2.* – www.competition-commission.org.uk/rep_pub/reports/2003/478vetmeds.htm (accessed 11 May 2007)

Department of Health (2000). *The NHS Plan: a plan for investment, a plan for reform.* www.dh.gov.uk/en/Publicationsandstatistics/Publications/PublicationsPolicyAndGuidance/DH_4002960

Crown Report (1998). *Review of prescribing, supply and administration of medicines. A report on the supply and administration of medicines under group prescribing.* (The first Crown report.) www.jcn. co.uk/pdf/crown report1.pdf (accessed 12 April 2007)

Crown Report (1999). *Review of prescribing, supply and administration of medicines. Final report (the second Crown report).* www.jcn.co.uk/pdf/ crownreport2.pdf (accessed 12th April 2007)

Royal Pharmaceutical Society of Great Britain (2007). *Medicines, Ethics and Practice Guide for Pharmacists and Pharmacy Technicians.* London: Pharmaceutical Press.

Useful resources

Drug Tariff: www.ppa.org.uk

General Dental Council register: www.gdc-uk.org/ Search+our+registers/Home.htm (accessed 24 April 2007)

General Medical Council List of registered medical practitioners: www.gmc-uk.org/register/index.asp

Office of Public Sector Information: www.opsi.gov.uk

Prescriptions Pricing Division: www.ppa.org.uk

10

Understanding and interpreting prescriptions

Sam E Weston

Introduction

This chapter describes in detail the FP10 – the prescription form use most frequently in England. It provides a thorough 'road map' to the details seen on such a form and also a comprehensive guide to interpreting the information presented on it. Before considering the prescription form and learning how to interpret it, some thought should be given to the whole prescribing process. Writing a prescription is only a small part of this process and there are several stages to go through – from diagnosis (defining the patient's problem), to choosing a suitable therapeutic objective (considering what needs to be treated), deciding on a suitable treatment regimen, prescribing the chosen regimen and, finally, monitoring the patient's progress.

The National Prescribing Centre (NPC) has developed seven principles of good prescribing for use in training supplementary prescribers (NPC, 1999), which have been adapted for the purposes of this chapter and are outlined in detail below.

Good prescribing principles – a stepwise approach

Figure 10.1 summarises the approach that should be adopted for good prescribing, the so-called pyramid. Each stage outlined in the diagram is explained below. Each step should be considered carefully before moving on to the next step.

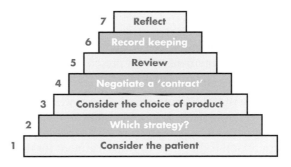

Figure 10.1   The prescribing pyramid. Each step should be considered carefully before continuing to the next step (NPC, 1999).

1 Examine the holistic needs of the patient

Is a prescription necessary? By first considering the holistic needs of the patient (such as their social and medical needs), early identification of non-drug therapy may become apparent, or perhaps the use of a complementary therapy in conjunction with mainstream medicinal therapy. Information such as the use of OTC medication or herbal or homoeopathic preparations should also be taken into account. Some patients will not divulge this information freely to their prescriber, or may not consider it relevant. Any details of previous drug allergies should also be confirmed.

Some pharmacists find mnemonics useful to help them remember the critical questions to ask patients during a consultation. (One example is the WWHAM approach, devised by the NPC, to remind pharmacists of five key points to cover when dispensing an OTC medication.). Bear in mind, however, that such mnemonics cannot be relied on to examine all pertinent areas required in each consultation.

2 Consider the therapeutic target

When a prescriber meets with a patient, it is important to bear in mind that other treatment options should be considered before writing a prescription. Some questions a prescriber must consider include:

- Has a diagnosis been made?
- Does the patient need a prescription at all?
- Are the patient's expectations a factor?

A prescription should only be given where there is a genuine need. It should also be remembered that patients may wish to receive a prescription for reasons other than to gain treatment for their condition (e.g. to legitimise the sick role, to gain attention, a friend has recommended it, or to get a prescription for a family member or friend).

3 Choosing a treatment and safety issues

The following issues should be explored when considering which product to prescribe.

- **How effective is the product?** To ensure that the most appropriate prescription item is selected, the prescriber needs to be familiar with the full range of items in the *British National Formulary* (*BNF*), or the formulary to which they are restricted. To assess how effective the product is, the available clinical evidence should be critically appraised. Websites such as the Department of Health's Research Findings Electronic Register (ReFeR; www.info.doh.gov.uk/doh/refr_web.nsf/home) give up-to-date information on recently developed, clinically trialled and newly released medicines. The National Library for Health (www.library.nhs.uk) provides information about treatment options for various illnesses.

- **How appropriate is the treatment?** Some drugs are contraindicated (unsuitable for use) in certain patients. For example, aspirin (or medicines containing it) should not be taken by patients with current or previous history of stomach ulcers, as it can irritate the stomach lining causing bleeding. The patient's medication history may also reveal potential drug interactions that may have serious consequences (e.g. warfarin and aspirin must not be taken together, because the combined anticoagulant effects of these two drugs may lead to an increased risk of bleeding).

In addition to choosing a product that is appropriate for the patient, the dose, formulation and duration of treatment should be tailored to the individual. Generally, an initial prescription should provide treatment for no more than 1 month, in order to ensure an early follow-up consultation to check on the patient's progress.

All drugs are associated with a certain risk of causing side-effects or adverse drug reactions (ADRs). ADRs account for 5% of all hospital admissions, and may be associated with a risk of significant morbidity and mortality (Pirmohamed *et al.*, 2004). The West Midlands Centre for Adverse Drug Reactions Studies website (www.adr.org.uk) provides up-to-date information on the incidence of ADRs. ADRs are also discussed in more detail in Chapter 6. For any given therapeutic intervention, the potential benefits of the treatment must always be balanced against safety concerns. The prescriber should be familiar with the common ADRs associated with the treatments they are prescribing.

4 Negotiate a 'contract' and achieve concordance with the patient

The prescriber and the patient should come to an understanding about the patient's illness and discuss potential treatments that will help the patient to reduce the effect it has on his/her life. Further information on concordance can be found in Chapter 14. Effective communication is an essential part of good practice (see Chapter 8) and includes the need to make sure that the patient understands the information given. In the case of prescribing a medicine, the patient needs to understand:

- what the medicine is for
- how to take the medicine
- at what dose and frequency to take it
- how long it takes to work
- how long to take the medicine for
- the possible side-effects and what to do if they occur.

5 Review the patient on a regular basis

Reviewing the patient enables the prescriber to establish whether the treatment prescribed is effective, safe and acceptable. In an ideal world, patients should be reassessed at least every 6 months, with no more than six repeat prescriptions given without review, as outlined in a comprehensive document produced by the NPC (2004). Repeat prescribing without proper review may be wasteful and inefficient, and may even be potentially dangerous in some cases.

6 Record keeping

Record keeping must be both accurate and up-to-date – comprehensive notes on the patient's

consultation, chosen drug regimen, test results and future appointments should be kept by the prescriber. In addition to this, the information recorded by the pharmacist (discussed in the following section) means a comprehensive record of the patient and their treatment is being maintained.

7 Reflection

This stage is often not considered until the patient returns for review with the prescriber. At this point the prescriber can decide whether the correct medicine regimen has been selected for the patient.

Interpretation of prescriptions

Once the prescription reaches you, the pharmacist, the next stage of the patient's care begins. To dispense a prescription, a methodical approach should be adopted in order to allow the prescriber's diagnosis and treatment choice to be conveyed accurately, with the correct medication, to the patient.

1 Check the patient's details

Firstly, the patient's details must be checked (see Figure 10.2). This allows the appropriateness of the treatment regimen for the particular patient to be assessed. Also, accurate records can be made of the product(s) dispensed, the product labelled for the patient, and the patient contacted, if necessary, after the medication has been dispensed and supplied to them. The full name of the patient is usually enough to indicate the sex of the patient, and therefore assess the appropriateness of a particular medication (e.g. finasteride should not be prescribed to women, except under certain circumstances when adequate contraceptive cover is in place, because it is highly toxic to developing male embryos).

The patient's address is also required (see Figure 10.2). This allows the pharmacist to

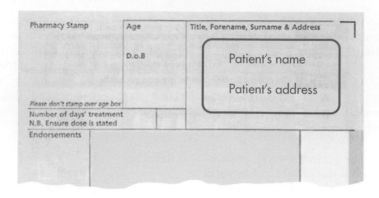

Figure 10.2 Check the patient's name (title, forename and surname) and address. The address is useful to distinguish between patients with the same name.

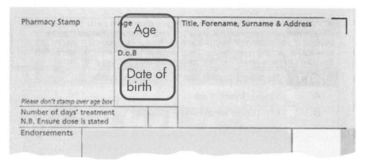

Figure 10.3 Check the patient's age and date of birth. The latter is useful to distinguish between patients with the same name and address. This information is also important to identify when the prescription is for a child.

distinguish between patients who may have the same name.

In the event that two patients have the same name and address, the date of birth (see Figure 10.3) should distinguish between them. This is also useful when calculation of appropriate dosages for children is required. It is a legal requirement for the date of birth to appear on an NHS prescription for children under the age of 12 years, but not on a private prescription.

2 Check the legal requirements of the prescription

The legal requirements are described in detail in Chapter 9; a summary is provided in Figures 10.4 and 10.5.

3 Check the product details

By checking the name of the drug prescribed, the required pharmaceutical form, the strength and the total amount to be dispensed, the pharmacist can check that they have sufficient quantity of the medicine in stock in their dispensary. Many medications are now available in 'patient packs' – a 28-day supply of medication in a box, complete with patient information leaflet – and it is not unusual for the prescriber to request '1 oP', meaning 'one original pack' is to be supplied. The quantity of medication to be supplied should be checked to ensure that the prescribed quantity is appropriate for the patient, as well as whether the medication is available in such a quantity. Some prescriptions are written to indicate that

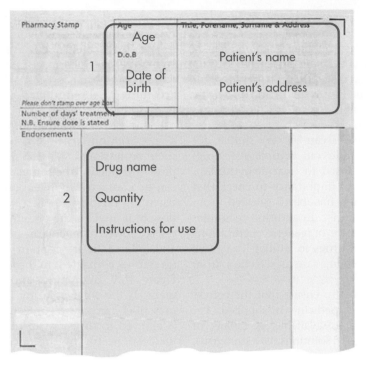

Figure 10.4   Legal requirements of the prescription, Part 1: (1) patient identification details; (2) details of prescribed medication.

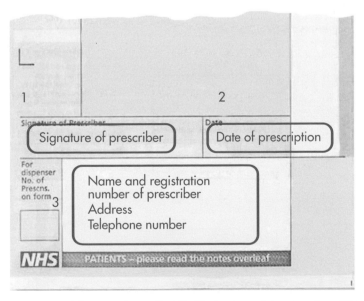

Figure 10.5   Legal requirements of the prescription, Part 2: (1) signature of the prescriber; (2) date before which the prescription cannot be dispensed; (3) prescriber's registration details.

a number of days' supply is to be provided (see Figure 10.6).

At this stage, the pharmacist should check that the medicine is available on the NHS (using the *Drug Tariff* as discussed in Chapter 9 or their computer labelling system), and also if the medication is available as a generic product or as a branded product.

Names of medicines can be very similar, for example dipyridamole (an antiplatelet drug) and disopyramide (used to treat arrhythmias), so it is of the utmost importance to check that the correct product has been selected from stock by the pharmacist. In addition to similar names, manufacturers of generic medications often package their drugs in similar livery (see Figure 10.7), so, again, careful selection from stock is required.

It is also important to ensure that the correct formulation of the medicine is supplied. For example, ibuprofen is available as tablets of different strengths, oral solutions (two strengths), oro-dispersible tablets, and gel for topical application to the skin (see Figure 10.8). In addition to this, if the medicine is available in different strengths, the pharmacist should ensure the correct strength has been selected from stock according to the information provided on the prescription.

In the event that information is missing from a prescription, the pharmacist should use their professional skills to decide whether the prescriber needs to be contacted. If the prescriber can be contacted by telephone for instructions regarding changes to the quantity, strength or dose indicated on the prescription, the pharmacist is allowed to amend the prescription by hand and endorse the prescription with the letters 'PC' (prescriber contacted) in the section indicated in Figure 10.9, and initial and date the amendment. If the total quantity is missing and the prescriber cannot be contacted, the pharmacist is allowed to dispense up to 5 days' supply of medication. In this instance the prescription

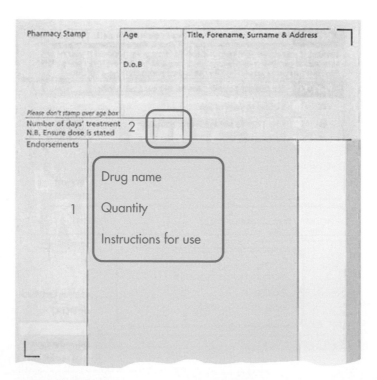

Figure 10.6   Check the details of the prescribed medication: name of drug, dosage form, strength (where appropriate) and either (1) quantity or (2) number of days' supply.

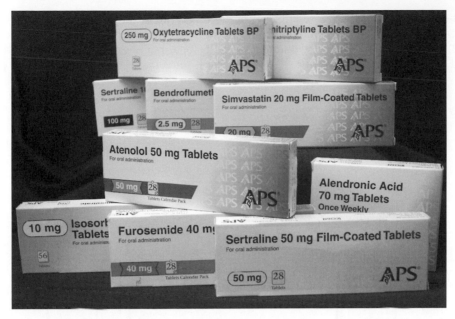

Figure 10.7   Check the name of the medication carefully. Generics manufacturers, in particular, provide a variety of medications in similar packaging.

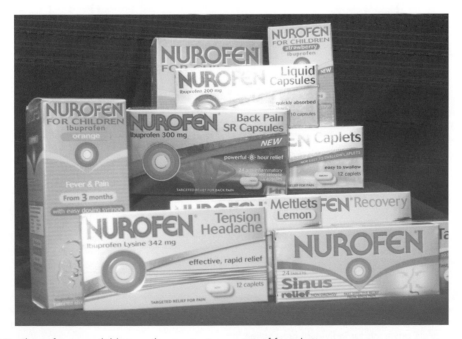

Figure 10.8   Ibuprofen is available over the counter in a variety of formulations.

should be endorsed 'PNC' (prescriber not contacted) and initialled and dated. Figure 10.9 (section 2) shows the area where the pharmacist is allowed to endorse the prescription.

4 Check the dosage and directions

The pharmacist should then check the dosage and directions for use of the prescribed

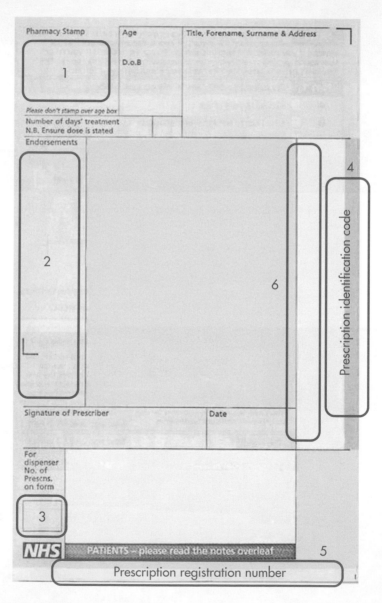

Figure 10.9   Endorsing guidelines: (1) details of the registered pharmacy premises; (2) details of medication(s) dispensed and any additional fees; (3) number of items dispensed. In addition, the prescription identifying code (4), and the unique prescription registration number (5) should be printed clearly. Section 6 is used by the Prescription Pricing Division to calculate payments for individual prescription forms.

medication. The dosage prescribed should always be checked with reference to the patient's age, as lower doses are often required in the case of children or elderly patients. Maximum doses and dosage regimens can be found in the *BNF* and *BNF for Children*. In the case of veterinary prescriptions, the dose and dosage regimen can be checked using the *Veterinary Pharmacopoeia* or in the Summary of product characteristics for veterinary medicines.

5 Check for interactions

The next important check to be made by the pharmacist is for potential interactions between medications. Many drugs are known to interact with each other; the most up-to-date source of information available to a pharmacist is Appendix 1 of the *BNF*. The *Pharmaceutical Journal*, which is the official weekly communication between the Royal Pharmaceutical Society of Great Britain (RPSGB) and all registered pharmacists, also provides regular updates on drug–drug interactions. All multiple-item prescriptions should be checked for potential interactions. If the patient's current medication record is available, this should also be checked for potential interactions between medications being supplied concurrently to the patient. If a particular prescribed medication is known to interact with many medications, OTC preparations or herbal medicines, the pharmacist should check with the patient which other medications they might be taking. All significant potential drug interactions should be referred to the prescriber. However, it is important to bear in mind that some interactions can be used therapeutically to enhance the effect of a prescribed medication. For example, diuretics increase the activity of some beta-blockers, so initially a lower dose of the latter is needed when the two drugs are used together in the treatment of hypertension (high blood pressure). The majority of prescription labelling systems (e.g. NexPhase, Enigma Healthcare) used in pharmacies have an inbuilt interaction alert system. However, pharmacists should be aware that they can vary in the accuracy and frequency with which they are updated; they are none the less a useful prompt to remind a pharmacist to look into some unusual interactions in more depth.

6 Produce a label

The labels for the medication give details of its name, strength, form and instructions for use. Labelling requirements are discussed in detail in Chapter 11. By producing these labels via the pharmacy's electronic patient medication record (PMR) system – used in conjunction with the electronic labelling system that generates labels for dispensed medications – the pharmacist is also automatically creating a record of the medication supplied to the patient.

7 Recording the prescription

Both legal and professional records of supply are needed. Professional records include PMRs; the types of data to record on such a system were defined by the RPSGB in 1996. An auditing procedure to ensure pharmacists adhere to these guidelines is available on the RPSGB website (www.rpsgb.org/pdfs/accuracy.pdf). Information should include:

- patient name, address (including postcode), and telephone number, age, date of birth, sex, NHS number
- prescriber information – name and identification number, practice details
- medicine supplied – name, strength, form and quantity, dosage regimen, date of dispensing
- patient exemption status, use of child-resistant closures, drug sensitivities, allergies, chronic illnesses.

Legal records required in the UK currently only extend to the maintenance of a private prescription register and controlled drug register. For private prescriptions, records are kept by hand in a bound book. Details recorded include:

- date of dispensing
- patient's name and address
- prescriber's details – address of practice, registration number

- prescribed medication – name, strength, form, quantity, directions for use
- price charged.

Note that information on price charged is not legally required but provides a useful reference for pharmacists in the event that the prescription is repeated. The private prescription charge may vary between pharmacies and depends on the cost of medication for the individual pharmacy and any 'mark up' on that cost, as well as professional charges for the pharmacist.

Controlled drugs

Controlled drug registers have been developed and enhanced over recent years, since the Shipman Inquiry (2004) called for closer monitoring of the supply of controlled drugs to prescribers and patients. Figure 10.10 shows an example of a partly completed recording sheet currently used in a community pharmacy environment, as supplied by the NPA.

Information recorded in the controlled drug register includes:

- name, brand (if applicable), strength and form of medication – currently one page is used per medication in order to keep records

separate from one another and enhance easier maintenance of stock levels
- date of transaction
- quantity of medication received into pharmacy stock
- address of supplier
- name and address of patient
- name and registration number of prescriber
- name and registration number of supplying pharmacist
- quantity of medication supplied
- identity of person collecting medication (type of identification seen, but this is not currently compulsory)
- running total of medication held in the controlled drugs cabinet.

8 The final check

Once the medication has been dispensed, the pharmacist (or an accredited checking technician) must carry out a final check which confirms all of the points discussed above for a second time. Where possible, the dispensing procedure and checking procedure should be carried out by a minimum of two people. This will help to reduce errors during the dispensing, labelling

Record of methadone oral solution 1 mg/mL			_S/F oral solution_					*
Date	**Obtained**		**Supplied**					**Balance**
	Name, address of person or firm from whom obtained	_Amount obtained_	_Name, address of person or firm supplied_	_Authority to possess – prescriber or licence holder details_	_Name and registration number of pharmacist supplying_	_Name of person collecting (and ID shown)_	_Amount supplied_	
02.02.07	AAH Pharmaceuticals, Invoice number	500 mL	-----------------------	-----------------------	--------------------	------------------	----------	500 mL
08.02.07	----------------------	---------	Mr Alan Simmons c/o Salvation Army	Dr S Smith 236752	Your surname Your registration number	Patient	10 mL	490 mL
*Insert details of formulation, eg 'sugar free', 'colour free' or solution made from powder or concentrate								

Figure 10.10   An example of a controlled drugs record sheet.

and checking of the prescribed medication, and ensure that the patient receives the correct medication, at the correct dose, in the correct form and with the correct directions for use.

9 Reimbursement

Once the final check has been performed, the prescription can be endorsed with exactly what was supplied to the patient so that the Prescription Pricing Division (PPD) can reimburse the pharmacy financially for the cost of the supplied medication. In addition, the pharmacist is currently paid a professional fee per item dispensed (applied to all items, including appliances).The current *Drug Tariff* gives the value for professional fees.

Additional fees are paid:

- when an item is dispensed extemporaneously – made up by the pharmacist on the pharmacy premises (e.g. aqueous cream with 1% menthol)
- for bulk prescriptions (e.g. medications supplied in large quantities for schools and institutions)
- for extra containers for extemporaneously dispensed liquids
- for controlled drugs
- for expensive items (PPD, 2007a).

The labelling programme may include an endorsement feature allowing the prescription to be endorsed electronically. NHS prescription forms are kept in the pharmacy for a month, before being sorted into categories defined by the PPD. The prescriptions are then packed and sent for processing (by no later than the fifth day of the month following that in which the medicine is dispensed) to one of ten PPDs – the processing arm of the NHS Business Services Authority (PPD, 2007b).

References

NPC (National Prescribing Centre) (1999). Signposts for prescribing nurses – general principles of good prescribing. *Prescribing Nurse Bulletin* 1: 1–4. www.npc.co.uk/nurse_prescribing/pdfs/signpostsvol1no1.pdf (accessed 12 April 2007).

NPC (National Prescribing Centre) (2004). *Saving time, helping patients: a good practice guide to quality repeat prescribing.* www.npc.co.uk/repeat_prescribing/pdf/repeat_prescribing_document1.pdf (accessed 20 December 2007).

Pirmohamed M, James S, Meakin S, *et al.* (2004). Adverse drug reactions as cause of admission to hospital: prospective analysis of 18 820 patients. *BMJ* 329:15–19.

PPD (Prescription Pricing Division) (2007a). *New Contractual Framework for Community Pharmacy; professional fees.* www.ppa.org.uk/ppa/contract_framework_for_community_pharmacy.htm#profees

PPD (Prescription Pricing Division) (2007b). *Processing and pricing.* www.ppa.org.uk/ppa/pro_price.htm

The Shipman Inquiry (2004). Chapter 7, Pharmacists and pharmacies; the controlled drugs register. In: *The fourth report – the regulation of controlled drugs in the community.* CM 6249. pp. 96–101. http://www.the-shipman-inquiry.org.uk/fourthreport.asp (accessed 20 December 2007).

Useful resources

Department of Health Research Findings Electronic Register (ReFeR): www.info.doh.gov.uk/doh/refr_web.nsf/Home

National Library of Health: www.library.nhs.uk

National Prescribing Centre: www.npc.co.uk

Pharmaceutical Journal

Prescription Pricing Division: www.ppa.org.uk

West Midland Centre for Adverse Drug Reactions: www.adr.org.uk

11

Packaging of medicines

Sam E Weston

Introduction

Medicines must be contained, protected and labelled appropriately, from the time of manufacture until the time they are used by a patient, in order to maintain their effectiveness as a medication, as well as allowing for accurate dispensing of the required dosage form, strength and quantity. After manufacture, the packaging of the medication must maintain the quality, safety and stability of the product and protect it from physical, climatic, chemical and biological hazards. Once the medication reaches the pharmacy, and is to be supplied to patients, the repackaged medicines should be easy to use and of a suitable size, in order to encourage patient adherence to their prescribed medication regimen. This chapter addresses the next stage of the dispensing procedure – that of choosing the correct packaging for the patient's medication once the dispensing procedure has begun.

Choice of packaging during dispensing

Several points need to be considered when selecting the correct packaging for your dispensed product.

The chemical nature of the product

Sensitivity to light, moisture and oxygen need to be considered, as well as compatibility with packaging materials. For example, glyceryl trinitrate tablets (used to treat angina) should always be supplied in a glass bottle because of the possibility of loss of the volatile drug and because it is soluble in some plastics. The lid of the bottle should be lined with aluminium foil, and the patient should be advised to keep the tablets at temperatures below 25°C. Even with all of these precautions in place, however, the tablets have a shelf life of only 8 weeks once the packaging has been opened.

Who will be taking the medication?

Elderly or arthritic patients may need non-child-resistant closures (CRC) or may want their medication to be dispensed into a monitored dosage system (MDS) box (see Figure 11.1). An MDS box is used to provide 1 week's medication in different time slots (breakfast, lunch, dinner and night). They are an essential means for some patients to retain their independence in medication taking.

Method of administration

Patients with insulin-dependent diabetes have to administer insulin by subcutaneous injection at specific times throughout the day in order to regulate their blood sugar. Insulin 'pens' allow patients to easily change the number of units of insulin they are injecting (see Figure 11.2).

Types of packaging

Packaging materials are divided into two categories – primary and secondary packaging –

and have different roles in the protection and delivery of the medication to the patient.

Primary packaging

Primary (or immediate) packaging is material that comes into direct contact with the medicine, which also includes the closure (defined as part of the primary packaging by the *British Pharmacopoeia* (*BP*) (BPC, 2007)). This material must protect the medicine from damage and from external interactions with chemical or biological sources. Primary packaging should also be convenient for patients, as described above.

Pharmacists have little choice in primary packaging materials, as most pharmaceutical products are now supplied by manufacturers in the correct packaging to ensure that product stability, safety and quality are maintained from the time of manufacture until the time of use by the patient.

Secondary packaging

Secondary packaging is additional material that improves the appearance of the medicine; it includes boxes, wrappers and labels that do not make direct contact with the dispensed product. These are often used to supply information to

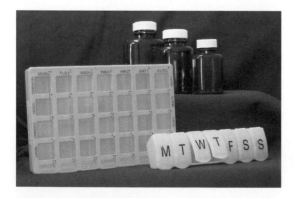

Figure 11.1 Non-child-resistant caps can be used on plastic dispensing bottles for elderly or arthritic patients. Elderly patients may also ask for their medicines to be dispensed in a monitored dosage system, two examples of which are shown here.

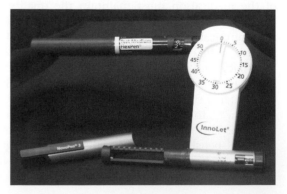

Figure 11.2 Three examples of insulin delivery pens; these allow patients to change the number of units they deliver.

Table 11.1   Definition of terms applied to packaging

Term	Definition	Example of use
Single dose	Containers hold a quantity of the preparation intended for total/partial use in a single administration	Preservative-free eye drops (Figure 11.3)
Multidose	Containers hold a quantity of preparation suitable for two or more repeated administrations	Injection (Figure 11.4)
Airtight	Containers are impenetrable to solids, liquids and gases under normal conditions of handling, storage and transport If intended to be opened more than once, the container must remain airtight after reclosure	Closure on a tub of cream/ointment (Figure 11.5)
Sealed	Containers are closed by fusion of the container material	Blister packs (Figure 11.6)
Tamper evident	Containers are closed and fitted with a device which reveals irreversibly that the container has been opened	Seal on creams before initial perforation (Figure 11.5)

Adapted from the *British Pharmacopoeia*, 2005

the patient about the product, and, as often as possible, clearly show if the packaged product has been tampered with.

different materials and defines several terms for use in the description of containers. Table 11.1 shows the most frequently used terms.

Definition of terms applied to packaging

Appendix XX of the *BP* (BPC, 2007) details the regulation of materials to be used in packaging of

Types of packaging materials

As mentioned in Chapter 12, some medication (mainly tablets and capsules) is packaged in patient packs. This is typically a 28-day supply

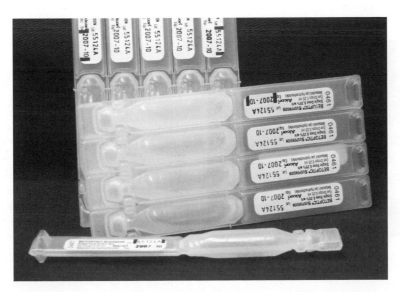

Figure 11.3   Single-dose vials of eye drops allow instillation of sterile drops at each point of administration.

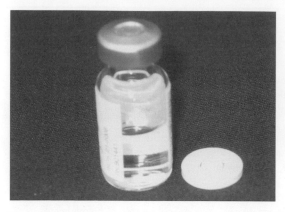

Figure 11.4   A multidose vial for repeated administration of the same medicine at different times.

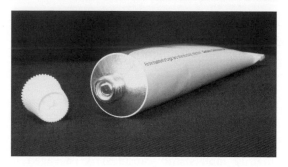

Figure 11.5   A tamper-evident seal; the metal container around the product is continuous until first administration by the patient, who breaks the seal using the point inside the cap.

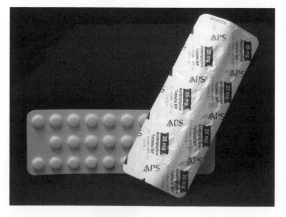

Figure 11.6   An example of a blister pack: tablets are held in individual moulded pockets on a plastic strip, heat sealed in place with a foil cover.

of medication and is often supplied in a blister pack (see Figure 11.6): the tablets are contained within a moulded plastic base layer and heat or pressure sealed with a thin foil layer. In addition, a patient information leaflet is supplied within the cardboard carton used to protect the blister pack. This combination of primary and secondary packaging is the most commonly seen when dispensing medicines. Other materials used for packaging are discussed below.

Paper

Paper has been used as a packaging material in pharmacy for longer than any other material. Although in modern day pharmacies paper is used largely as a secondary packaging material as a carton to hold the primary packaging material, early medicines of dried herbs or minerals such as chalk were powdered and supplied in paper packets. Indeed, paper has also been used as part of the dosage form – unpleasant tasting powders were sometimes taken wrapped in a rice-paper wafer, softened by dipping in water, then swallowing with a draught of water. This idea was further developed in France by Limousin of Paris in the 1870s with the *cachet*, two rice-paper cups which were joined together with powder inside; the early ancestor of the capsule (RPSGB, 2007a).

Glass

Glass has been widely used as a primary packaging material and is particularly useful for liquid formulations, as it is rigid, has superior protective qualities and allows for easy inspection of the contents. It is also impermeable to air and moisture, does not react with most medicinal products, and can be coloured in order to protect the contents from light when required. Moreover, it is easy to clean, can be sterilised by heat and even sealed to completely enclose a dosage form (e.g. injection liquids; see Figure 11.7). Glass for medicinal packaging is currently divided into four main categories defined by the *European Pharmacopoeia* (Council of Europe, 1991).

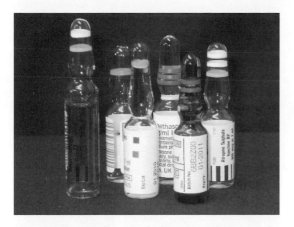

Figure 11.7 A selection of glass ampoules; ampoules are sealed by heat fusing Type I glass, producing a single unit dose that is protected from air and moisture. Coloured glass is used to protect light-sensitive medications.

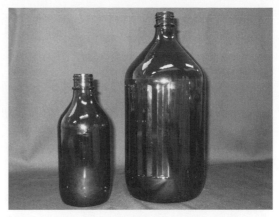

Figure 11.8 Examples of Winchester dispensing bottles; pharmacists can dispense the volume of liquid prescribed from these bulk-packed medications.

- **Type I – neutral or borosilicate glass.** This is the least chemically reactive type of glass and also does not expand or crack on exposure to temperature changes. It is used mainly to package fluids for injection.
- **Type II – sodalime-silicate glass.** This type is chemically treated so that the inside surface is as unreactive as Type I glass. It is used largely to produce containers for eye, ear and nasal drops. This type of glass may react with chemicals in the medicines and it is recommended they are used only once before disposal, because of the possibility of breakdown of the internal surface layer.
- **Type III – sodalime-silicate glass.** This is similar in composition to Type II glass, but has lower alkali content. It contains some chemicals that may leach (move out of the glass) into the preparation it contains. It is used to package liquids dispensed from Winchester bottles (large volumes of liquid drug formulations) (see Figure 11.8) in pharmacies. Although it is of a lower quality than Types I and II glass, it is much cheaper to produce and is therefore ideal for the quick turnover of large-volume liquid products.
- **Type IV – sodalime-silicate glass.** This glass is also similar in composition to Types II and III, but has even higher capability to leach chemicals into the contained product. It should not be used to package materials for injection, but is suitable for packaging solids (tablets) and semisolid formulations (creams, ointments).

Types of glass container commonly used in the pharmacy

- **Bottles** can be amber metric medical bottles or ribbed oval bottles. Amber bottles are used to package a wide range of oral medications. Ribbed (or fluted) bottles are used to package medicinal products that should not be taken orally (e.g. menthol and eucalyptus inhalation) and were traditionally used to dispense poisons. Historically, poison bottles were distinguishable by touch by attaching sandpaper to the surface, by painting thick lines on the outer surface or even by attaching bells to them (RPSGB, 2007b). Preparations to be dispensed in ribbed bottles are listed in section 1.2.7 of *Medicines, Ethics and Practice Guide for Pharmacists and Pharmacy Technicians*. Pharmacists are advised to refer to this list in the event of dispensing medicines into a bottle, as it is updated every 6 months. Figure 11.9 shows some of the glass dispensing bottles commonly in use today.
- **Dropper bottles** (see Figure 11.10) are used to contain medicinal products for application to the eye, ear or nose, and are usually hexagonal and fluted on three sides. They are fitted

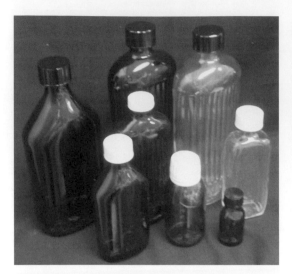

Figure 11.9   Glass dispensing bottles come in a range of sizes. Amber bottles are used for medicinal products that are light-sensitive; clear bottles can be used for those that are not light-sensitive. Ribbed or fluted bottles are used for medicinal products that should not be taken orally. Bottles can be closed with child-resistant closures or normal caps.

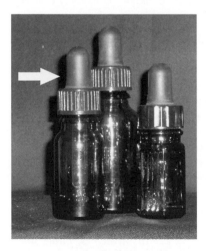

Figure 11.10   Dropper bottles for eye, ear or nose drops. The arrow indicates the combination cap closure used in many dropper bottles, composed of a plastic screw thread cap, a rubber teat and the glass dropper.

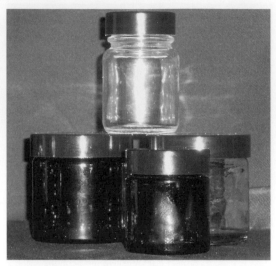

Figure 11.11   Jars for creams and ointments.

patients' fingers will not affect the product stability.

- **Ampoules** (see Figure 11.7). Single-use injections are often supplied in ampoules, in either liquid or powder form. The neck of the ampoule provides a weak area where the glass can be snapped easily, allowing either withdrawal of the solution by syringe, or addition of a diluent in the case where the ampoule contents require reconstitution before administration.
- **Multidose vials** (see Figure 11.4) are used to store injection solutions that will be used more than once. They are usually sealed with a rubber plug that is held in place by an aluminium sealing ring (Winfield & Richards, 2003).The bung is made of special material that can be pierced by needle many times, without any loss of sealing properties, allowing for continued protection against moisture and bacteria.

Plastic

Plastics have been widely used for several years as primary and secondary packaging for medicines. They come in many forms, including rigid bottles that loose tablets and capsules are dispensed into, squeezable bottles for eye drops and nasal sprays, jars, sachets, blister packs, and

with a combined cap, rubber teat and dropper as the closure mechanism.

- **Jars** (see Figure 11.11). Creams and ointments are supplied in wide-mouthed cylindrical jars in situations where contamination from infusion bags for the delivery of large volumes of fluid intravenously. Plastics are resistant to breakage and can be made opaque in order to protect light-sensitive medications. They are divided into two classes: thermosets and thermoplastics. Thermoset plastics are used for screw caps for glass and metal containers. Thermoplastics are used for packaging such as rigid bottles (see Figure 11.1), flexible eye-drop bottles, heat-sealable containers (as used to seal some types of MDS), intravenous solution bags and bottles, and containers for oils and creams.

Metal

Metal is often used in the form of a collapsible metal tube as a primary packaging material for creams and ointments. The tubes are made from aluminium, which remains collapsed as the product is used by the patient.

Aluminium foil is used in blister packaging (see Figure 11.6) to form a moisture-impermeable barrier that protects tablets and capsules held in plastic strips. Strip packaging of medicines sensitive to light and moisture involves sealing each individual dosage unit (tablet or capsule) in a foil 'pouch' on a strip of 7–10 units. This individual wrapping of the medicine protects the medicine from exposure to light and/or moisture, which cause breakdown of the drug. Epilim tablets (which contain the anticonvulsant sodium valproate, used to treat epilepsy) are packaged in this way.

Closures

Closures are defined as part of medicines packaging material by the BP. They should provide an effective seal to retain the dispensed medications within the packaging, and also protect the contents from contamination. The majority of loose medication dispensed from a bulk supply provided by a manufacturer is packaged into a plastic or glass bottle with a CRC (the most common 'push down and turn' cap is known as a 'Clic Loc'). Use of a CRC is a professional requirement for dispensing solid and liquid medications in the UK, but should not be considered as an absolute barrier to children. Patients should always be advised to store medications in a safe place that is out of the reach and sight of children.

Other closures include the rubber stopper used to seal multidose injection vials, which reseals after perforation by a needle. It can also undergo heat sterilisation – once the medication has been placed into the vial by the manufacturer and the rubber stopper inserted, the complete package is usually heat sterilised in order to remove any bacterial contamination.

Environmental concerns

Packaging is obviously a necessity in order to allow safe transport and storage of medications from the manufacturer, via wholesalers, on to dispensaries and ultimately to the patient. It has a negative impact on the environment in its consumption of raw materials and energy during production, and ends up as waste material requiring suitable disposal. As yet, there is no requirement or facility in place for pharmacies to dispose of pharmaceutical packaging.

Under the third essential service of the new Pharmacy Contract (see Chapters 3 and 6), every pharmacy must provide facilities for the disposal of unwanted medicines. Pharmacists should remind patients to bring back unused medications to the pharmacy for safe disposal. Unwanted medicines are disposed of via pharmaceutical waste specialists, contracted to the local health authority.

Practicalities of packaging

A large proportion of medicines that pass through a pharmacy will require repackaging in some way. Patient packs are the exception to this. Blister-packed tablets may need dispensing into appropriately sized cartons; bulk liquids will need decanting into bottles of different volumes; bulk quantities of loose tablets and capsules will be transferred into plastic bottles of a variety of sizes.

Factors to consider when choosing packaging

Pharmacists need to consider many factors when choosing packaging materials for medicines dispensing.

Patient needs

The majority of patients will be able to use blister packs or CRC bottles with few problems. However, consider use by elderly patients or those with poor manual dexterity; these patients may need you to transfer the tablets or capsules from the blister packs into an MDS or simply into a plastic bottle with a non-CRC lid. However, pharmacists must then consider how the stability of the tablets may be affected – changing the storage conditions of some medicines may make them unsuitable for use for patients. For example, controlled-release sodium valproate tablets (Epilim, used to treat epilepsy) interact with moisture in the air as soon as they are exposed to the atmosphere and within a week contain a subtherapeutic dose of medication. In this situation, patients should be advised not to take tablets that have been opened for more than 7 days.

If repackaging a medicine, choose appropriately sized packaging. If the prescription requires only a few tablets or capsules that are in a blister pack, then choose a suitable sized dispensing carton to package them in. A small number of tablets or capsules in a large box may possibly rattle around, causing mechanical damage to the dosage form and possible rendering them unsuitable for use. A prescription asking for 100 mL calamine lotion should be dispensed into the appropriately sized bottle, which is both easier to transport and easier for the patient to use when administering the lotion.

During the final packaging procedure, after the medication has been checked against the prescription, the pharmacist should carefully pack the medication into a dispensing bag, ensuring that the bag bears the correct patient's name. Placing medicine in the wrong bag could result in a patient taking the wrong medication, with potentially disastrous consequences. Remember to make the bag as anonymous as possible. It is vital to consider patient confidentiality at all times; patients may not want other people to know that they have medication, or what it may be for.

References

BPC (British Pharmacopoeia Commission) 2007. *British Pharmacopoeia*. London: Stationery Office.

Council of Europe (1991). *European Pharmacopoeia: 6th edition.* Luxembourg: 2007.

RPSGB (Royal Pharmaceutical Society of Great Britain) (2007a). Powders and cachets. Information sheet 8. www.rpsgb.org/pdfs/mussheet08.pdf (accessed 1 May 2007).

RPSGB (Royal Pharmaceutical Society of Great Britain) (2007b). Dispensary bottles. Information sheet 12. www.rpsgb.org/pdfs/mussheet12.pdf (accessed 1 May 2007).

Winfield A J, Richards R M E (2003). *Pharmaceutical Practice,* 3rd edn. Edinburgh: Churchill Livingstone.

Useful resources

British Pharmacopoeia Commission; provides online access to the full text of the *British Pharmacopoeia* for registered users and links to other national pharmacopeias and regulatory agencies. www.pharmacopoeia.org.uk

Royal Pharmaceutical Society of Great Britain (2007). *Medicines, Ethics and Practice Guide for Pharmacists and Pharmacy Technicians,* 31st edn. London: Pharmaceutical Press.

12

Labelling of medicines

Sam E Weston

Introduction

This chapter introduces labelling of medicinal products; at this stage the pharmacist needs to clearly pass on directions for use from the prescriber to the patient. Apart from the many legal issues surrounding medications and labelling requirements, you should by now realise the importance of communicating accurate information to patients. The information summarised on a label is available to the patient every time they take a dose of a medicine. In addition to covering requirements for dispensing labels, this chapter also addresses the legal (UK and European Union) and professional requirements for the labelling of medicinal products:

- dispensed medications
- pre-packed bulk medications
- chemists' nostrums
- manufacturers' labels
- medicines: general sales list (GSL), pharmacy-only (P) and prescription-only medicines (POM)
- veterinary-prescribed medications.

Containers of medicinal products sold or supplied in the UK must be labelled in accordance with the Medicines (Marketing Authorisations and Miscellaneous Amendments) Regulations 1994 (OPSI, 2004). Medicinal products classified as Schedule 2 or 3 controlled drugs must also be labelled in accordance with the Misuse of Drugs Regulations 2001 (OPSI, 2001). The *Medicines, Ethics and Practice Guide for Pharmacists and Pharmacy Technicians* provides the most recently published information regarding the categorisation of medicines and changes to labelling requirements (RPSGB, 2007).

The primary purpose of good labelling is defined by the Medicines and Healthcare products Regulatory Agency (MHRA) (2002) as '. . . the clear unambiguous identification of the medicine and the conditions for its safe use'.

The importance of labelling

Labels are an important factor to consider in the final presentation of a medication that will be released to a patient. A clearly worded,

117

professionally finished label, which is affixed in line with the edges of the container or package of the medication, will give the patient confidence that the preparation of the medication has been handled in a professional manner.

A label can be considered as a mechanism for passing on information from the physician to the patient in the event of the medicine being prescribed. It is used to identify who the medication is for (patient's name), what the product is (drug name, strength and pharmaceutical form), the date it was dispensed to the patient and as an *aide memoir* in how to take the medication correctly (directions for use).

In the event the product has been passed from manufacturer to the pharmacist, labels on original packaging materials contain identifying details of the product stored within the container, its date of expiry and licensing details.

From this, it can be seen that accurate labelling is of the utmost importance. The MHRA's *Best practice guidance on labelling and packaging of medicines* covers current labelling requirements in depth (MHRA, 2007).

Labelling requirements for different categories of medicinal products

All labels must be written indelibly; the majority are now computer generated and should there-fore be easily legible. The following section describes the information required on labels for different classes of medicines.

Dispensed medicinal products

A dispensed medicinal product is defined in several ways:

- a product prepared or dispensed by a pharmacist
- a product prepared or dispensed by a physician or prepared or dispensed in accordance with a prescription supplied by a physician
- a product for use by human beings supplied by a doctor or dentist to a particular patient under their care, or to a representative of the patient (e.g. a parent or carer).

The labelling requirements for such medicinal products are found in the Medicines (Marketing Authorisations and Miscellaneous Amendments) Regulations 1994 (as amended in 2004). An adapted list of the legal requirements is provided in Box 12.1 (see also Figures 12.1 and 12.2).

The pharmacist should also take care with the wording of instructions on the label. The Royal Pharmaceutical Society of Great Britain has published a Working Party Report which made several recommendations regarding the way in which directions for use should be worded

---

Box 12.1 The legal requirements for labelling of medicinal products

- name of patient
- name and address of supplier (usually the dispensing pharmacy registered premises)
- Date dispensed
- the phrase 'Keep out of reach and sight of children'*
- name, strength and pharmaceutical formulation of the product
- directions for use, such as 'Shake the bottle before use' for liquids or suspensions
- the phrase 'For external use only' within a box if the medication is not a general sales list

medication and is an embrocation, liniment, lotion, liquid antiseptic or other liquid preparation or gel that is for external use only
- warning labels – these are usually produced automatically by the electronic labelling software used to prepare labels for dispensed medications; a list of these can be found at the back of the *British National Formulary* in abbreviated form or in Appendix 9 in their full form

* Note that 'and sight' is added as good practice but is not a legal requirement

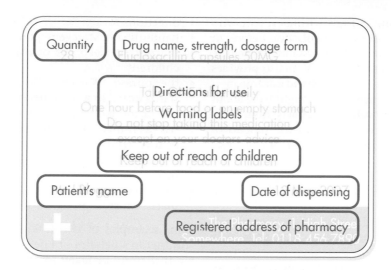

Figure 12.1   An example of a dispensing label, showing the layout of information seen on most labels on dispensed medication.

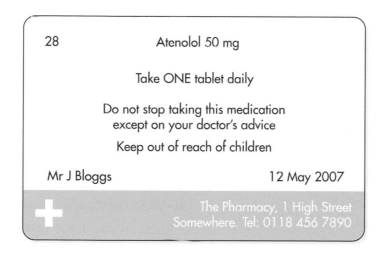

Figure 12.2   A sample dispensing label for a medicinal product. The information is clear and concise for the patient to understand easily.

(RPSGB, 2001). For example, 'take' is more easily understood by patients than 'to be taken'; 'apply' is preferred to 'to be applied'. Also, the recommended directions for taking tablets and capsules are: 'Take one tablet/capsule twice each day' (rather than 'Take one twice daily'). Research has shown that inserting the dosage form between the number of dosage units to be taken (one), and the frequency of administration (twice) ensured the patient did not mix up the two numbers. Finally, the importance of verbally communicating the information provided on the label directly to the patient should not be underestimated. Best practice guidelines suggest that a pharmacist should consult with a patient who has not taken a particular medication before, in order to ensure that they understand how to take the medication. This consultation also provides the patient with the opportunity to ask any questions about any concerns they might have about their illness or possible side-effects from their medication, and contributes to the process of concordance (discussed in Chapter 14).

Prepacked bulk medications

As mentioned in Chapter 11, some medicines are packaged by manufacturers in large bulk containers, which are then used as stock from which pharmacists dispense. In some dispensaries these bulk stocks are packed down into more easily handled amounts for dispensing against prescriptions – a term known as 'assembly'. Medicines repackaged in this way require labels to contain the following information:

- name of product
- ingredients of product
- quantity in container
- special requirements with regard to handling or storage
- expiry date
- batch number (starting with the letters 'BN').

Before dispensing to a patient, these medicines must be relabelled according to the requirements for dispensed medications (Box 12.1).

Chemists' nostrums

A 'nostrum' is rather unflatteringly defined in the *Oxford English Dictionary* as a 'quack remedy or patent medicine, usually of secret ingredient, with unproven efficacy'. The preparation of chemists' nostrums, which remain popular with many patients, and their sale or supply must be carried out under the supervision of a pharmacist. The label of the container of these medicinal products must show the following details:

- name of the product
- the pharmaceutical form: ingredients – including concentrations and strengths – and quantity

- directions for use
- handling and storage requirements
- the phrase 'Keep out of reach and sight of children'
- the phrase 'Warning. Do not exceed the stated dose.' in a box (this is necessary where one or more of the ingredients is a POM that has been used in such a way as to allow it to be used without POM restrictions)
- the name and address of the registered pharmacy
- the letter 'P' in a box (to indicate that a pharmacist must be present when it is dispensed).

Some examples of chemists' nostrums include 'Turlington's Balsalm of Life' – an alleged 'cure-all' that could be taken internally or rubbed on to affected parts of the body to relieve pain in the joints, and 'Robertson's Infallible Worm Destroying Lozenges' – which could be used at one dose by humans and at a higher dose for treating horses.

Manufacturers' labelling requirements

The labelling requirements for manufactured medications are comprehensive and are defined by the Medicines (Marketing Authorisations and Miscellaneous Amendments) Regulations 1994 (as amended in 2004). Figure 12.3 shows a sample of the information that would be contained on a manufacturer's bulk supply of a POM. At the time of writing the legal requirements include:

- name, strength and pharmaceutical form of the medicine
- ingredients – quantities of each excipient included in the dosage unit
- quantity of product – by weight, volume or number of doses contained within the packaging
- a list of all excipients with a known pharmacological effect
- the method or route of administration of the product
- warning 'keep out of reach and sight of children'
- any special warnings required by the marketing authorisation for the product concerned

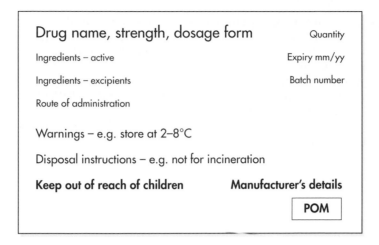

Figure 12.3   An example of the information required on a manufacturer's label for the bulk supply of a prescription-only medicine (POM).

- the expiry date of the product, clearly stating month and year
- any special storage details
- any information about special disposal requirements
- name and address detail of the market authorisation holder and any number as allocated by the licensing authority
- manufacturer's batch reference.

Manufacturers are also encouraged to label products with a summary of product characteristics, useful for health education purposes. Labelling of a promotional nature is not permitted. In addition these labels must contain information presented in a legible format that is easily understood by all of those involved in its supply and use, and this information must be in English (and one or more additional languages; the same information must be reproduced in all languages used).

General sales list products

Medicinal products that are available as GSL products (i.e. sold in other retail outlets in addition to pharmacies) and that contain aloxiprin, paracetamol or aspirin require the following labels on the packaging:

- if containing aloxiprin, paracetamol or aspirin, the words 'If symptoms persist, consult your doctor' and details of the recommended dosage
- if containing aloxiprin, the words 'Contains an aspirin derivative'
- if containing aspirin, the words 'Contains aspirin'
- if containing aloxiprin or aspirin, the words 'Do not give to children under the age of 16 years, unless on the advice of a doctor' – aspirin and its derivatives are not recommended for children under 16 years of age because of an association with Reye's syndrome; this information should also be contained on the patient information leaflet (PIL)
- if containing paracetamol, the words 'Contains paracetamol'
- if the medicine is paracetamol-based and is intended to be used for children under 12 years of age, the warnings 'Do not give with any other paracetamol-containing product' and 'Immediate medical advice should be sought in the event of an overdose, even if the child seems well, because there is a risk of delayed, serious liver damage' – the latter part of this information can be contained on the PIL one is supplied with the product
- if the medicine is paracetamol-based and intended to be used for adults, the warnings

'Do not take with any other paracetamol-containing product' and 'Immediate medical advice should be sought in the event of an overdose, even if you feel well, because there is a risk of delayed, serious liver damage'; the latter part of this information can be contained on the PIL if one is supplied with the product

- any product containing paracetamol should carry the label 'Do not exceed the stated dose', positioned next to the dosage instructions.

Pharmacy medicines

Medicinal products for sale as 'P' medicines (for sale only under the supervision of a pharmacist), must carry the following labels on the packaging:

- the packaging must contain the letter 'P' in a box
- if the medicinal product contains aloxiprin, aspirin or paracetamol, the same labelling requirements that apply to GSL medicines apply
- if the product contains a POM in a quantity that allows it to be exempt from POM controls, the label 'Warning. Do not exceed the stated dose' must be on the packaging
- if the product contains ephedrine (or any of its salts), or is to be used for the treatment of asthma or conditions associated with bronchial spasm, the label 'Warning. Asthmatics should consult their doctor before using this product' should be on the packaging
- products containing ingredients that may cause drowsiness should be labelled with the phrase 'Warning. May cause drowsiness. If affected do not drive or operate machinery. Avoid alcoholic drinks'
- any embrocation, liniment, lotion, liquid antiseptic or other liquid preparation or gel for use on the skin should contain the label 'For external use only'
- products containing hexachlorophane (e.g. some alcohol-free hand sanitisers) must be labelled with the phrase 'Not to be used for babies' or a warning that it should not be used

in children under 2 years of age (hexachlorophane has the potential to cause brain damage during the early stages of child development).

Prescription-only medicines

Many of the labelling requirements for POMs have been addressed in earlier sections of this chapter. In addition, packaging should contain the following labels:

- the letters 'POM' in a box
- 'For external use only' if the medication is to be used on the surface of the skin
- if the product contains hexachlorophane, the warning label 'Not to be used for babies' or a warning that the product is not to be administered to children under 2 years of age.

Veterinary products

In 2002 the Competition Commission published a report on veterinary medicines which outlined a monopoly situation in which veterinarians were prescribing and supplying medicines to owners of pets. Recommendations have therefore been made to encourage the supply of veterinary medications from pharmacies, and pharmacists are increasingly being presented with veterinary prescriptions. Containers of medicines dispensed for animal use must show:

- the name of the person controlling the animal/herd
- the address of the location where the animal/herd resides or the named person's address
- the name and address of the supplier
- date dispensed
- directions for use
- the phrase 'Keep out of the reach and sight of children'
- the phrase 'for animal treatment only'
- at the request of the veterinary surgeon, the label should contain details of:
  - product name
  - directions for use
  - precautions.

In the event that the medicinal product is being supplied in bulk form, containers of medicines supplied for animal use must show:

- product name
- quantities of various ingredients
- quantity of dosage units supplied
- directions for use
- contraindications, warnings and precautions
- the phrases 'For animal treatment only' and 'Keep out of reach and sight of children'
- an appropriate withdrawal period before slaughter (if necessary)
- handling and storage requirements
- expiry date
- marketing authorisation number
- batch reference number
- manufacturer's name and address
- species of animal for which it is to be used
- legal classification (e.g. 'P', POM, pharmacy and merchants' list (PML), GSL, medicated feedingstuff medicine (MFS), MFS exempted from prescription-only status (MFSX)
- any further information required by the marketing authorisation licence.

Other labelling requirements

In the event that a medication is dispensed using emergency supply procedures, the words 'Emergency supply' must appear on the label. The *Medicines, Ethics and Practice Guide for Pharmacists and Pharmacy Technicians* provides details of the procedure to be followed when a medication is supplied on an emergency supply basis. In the case of a private prescription being dispensed, a reference number corresponding to the relevant entry in the private prescriptions register should appear on the label.

Practicalities of labelling

The following factors should be considered with dispensed medications – the area in which the pharmacist has the most influence in labelling medicinal products.

- Who will read the label: Is their vision impaired? Do they read English? Translations of many patient information leaflets are available to the pharmacist (for printing) from manufacturers' websites. The Royal National Institute for the Blind Medicine Information Line (http://xpil.medicines.org. uk/RNIBInfo; telephone 0800 198 5000) provides patient information leaflets in large clear format or Braille; in addition, patients can have a patient information leaflet read to them over the telephone.
- Where will the label will be placed? Don't obscure important manufacturer's information (e.g. expiry date, storage conditions, etc.).
- Which part of the medicine will be labelled? For example, for ointments, creams and inhalers, should the label go on the tube or the box? Best practice suggests double labelling of products that come in an external package, so that both the box and the item inside are labelled, in order to ensure that patients retain a label with instructions even if they discard external packaging.

References

Competition Commission (2002). *Veterinary Medicines: A report on the supply within the United Kingdom of prescription-only veterinary medicines Volumes 1 & 2.* – www.competition-commission. org.uk/rep_pub/reports/2003/478vetmeds.htm (accessed 11 May 2007).

Medicines and Healthcare products Regulatory Agency (MHRA) (2002). www.mhra.gov.uk (accessed 8 May 2007).

Medicines and Healthcare products Regulatory Agency (MHRA) (2007). Labels, patient information leaflets and packaging for medicines. www.mhra.gov.uk/home/idcplg?IdcService=SS_GET_ PAGE&nodeId= 164 (accessed 9 May 2007).

Office of Public Sector Information (OPSI) (2001). Statutory Instrument 2001 No. 3998. The Misuse of Drugs Regulations 2001. www.opsi.gov.uk/si/si2001/20013998.htm (accessed 8 May 2007).

Office of Public Sector Information (OPSI) (2004). Statutory Instrument 2004 No. 3224. The Medicines

(Marketing Authorisations and Miscellaneous Amendments) Regulations 2004. www.opsi.gov.uk/si/si2004/20043224.htm (accessed 8 May 2007).

Royal Pharmaceutical Society of Great Britain (RPSGB) (2001). *The Way Forward in the New Millennium. Report of the Royal Pharmaceutical Society's Working Party on Drug Delivery*. www.rpsgb.org/pdfs/sciwp drugdel-i.pdf (accessed 9 May 2007).

Royal Pharmaceutical Society of Great Britain (RPSGB) (2007). *Medicines, Ethics and Practice Guide for Pharmacists and Pharmacy Technicians*, 31st edn. London: Pharmaceutical Press.

13

Extemporaneous dispensing: a beginner's guide

Sam E Weston and Kate E Fletcher

What is extemporaneous dispensing?

The word 'extemporaneous' is derived from the Latin *'ex tempore'* meaning 'on the spur of the moment'. The *Oxford English Dictionary* definition is 'spoken or done without preparation' (Oxford University Press, 2005). In pharmacy, it refers to the preparation of small quantities of a medicine from its constituent ingredients (Winfield & Richards, 2004).

Most pharmaceutical products are now made in large-scale manufacturing facilities, with high standards of quality assurance. It is not possible for individual pharmacies to match these standards and so it is preferable for a licensed medicine to be prescribed and dispensed from commercial stocks rather than for an extemporaneous preparation to be made. Indeed, the *Medicines, Ethics and Practice Guide for Pharmacists and Pharmacy Technicians* specifies that a licensed product must always be prescribed and dispensed *when one is available*. It is nevertheless important that pharmacists learn and maintain the skills required to make extemporaneous preparations, or 'extemps', as they are often referred to. This chapter describes some of the techniques used in the manufacture of some relatively commonplace extemporaneous preparations: oral liquids (e.g. suspensions and syrups) and topical semisolids (e.g. creams and ointments).

Legal factors involved in extemporaneous preparation

Standards for extemporaneous preparation and compounding are set out in the *Medicines, Ethics and Practice Guide for Pharmacists and Pharmacy Technicians*, and are outlined in Box 13.1.

Where possible, all calculations and measurements should be double checked by a second appropriately trained member of staff, except where methadone mixture is prepared extemporaneously in accordance with Appendix 1 (available at www.rpsgb.org.uk/protectingthepublic/ethics/).

The *Medicines, Ethics and Practice Guide for Pharmacists and Pharmacy Technicians* (RPSGB, 2007) should be consulted for the most current legal guidelines, which are often subject to change or amendment.

Box 13.1 Extemporaneous preparation or compounding standards as set out in the *Medicines, Ethics and Practice Guide for Pharmacists and Pharmacy Technicians*

This standard is not intended to cover the reconstitution of dry powders with water or other diluents. Patients are entitled to expect that products prepared extemporaneously in a pharmacy are prepared accurately and are suitable for use. If you wish to be involved in extemporaneous preparation you must ensure the following.

1. A product is extemporaneously prepared only when there is no product with a marketing authorisation available and where you are able to prepare the product in compliance with accepted standards.
2. You and any other staff involved are competent to undertake the tasks to be performed.
3. The requisite facilities and equipment are available. Equipment must be maintained in good order to ensure that performance is unimpaired, and must be fit for the intended purpose.
4. You are satisfied as to the safety and appropriateness of the formula of the product.
5. Ingredients are sourced from recognised pharmaceutical manufacturers and are of a quality accepted for use in the preparation and manufacture of pharmaceutical products. Where appropriate, relevant legislation must be complied with.

6. Particular attention and care is paid to substances which may be hazardous and require special handling techniques.
7. The product is labelled with the necessary particulars, including an expiry date and any special requirements for the safe handling or storage of the product.
8. If you are undertaking large-scale preparation of medicinal products, all relevant standards and guidance are adhered to.
9. Records are kept for a minimum of 2 years. The records must include:

    - the formula
    - the ingredients
    - the quantities used
    - their source
    - the batch number
    - the expiry date
    - where the preparation is dispensed in response to a prescription, the patient's and prescription details and the date of dispensing
    - the personnel involved, including the identity of the pharmacist taking overall responsibility.

Liquid preparations

Oral liquids

An oral liquid is a preparation containing one or more active ingredients in a suitable vehicle and is intended to be swallowed (Lund, 1994). The three main types of oral liquids are solutions, suspensions and emulsions. A few oral liquids may be a pure liquid that is the active constituent (e.g. liquid paraffin).

Advantages of oral liquids

Oral liquids are generally easier to swallow than a solid dosage form such as a tablet or capsule, and the active constituent is absorbed more rapidly from the gastrointestinal tract. Liquids can be particularly useful for children, the elderly, and patients with conditions such as Parkinson's disease because of relative ease of taking the preparation.

Disadvantages of oral liquids

Bottles of liquid can be bulky and heavy and are therefore less portable than tablets and capsules. Glass bottles are also prone to breaking if not handled carefully. It is more difficult to mask the unpleasant taste of some medications in a liquid than in a solid dosage form, and liquids are less stable, both microbiologically and chemically (Lund, 1994). The liquid must be measured carefully by the patient to ensure the correct dose is taken, which some patients might find difficult, particularly if they have conditions that affect manual dexterity, such as rheumatoid arthritis.

Oral solutions

There are several different types of oral solutions (Lund, 1994; Winfield & Richards, 2004).

- **An elixir** is a clear flavoured liquid that contains one or more active ingredients dissolved in a vehicle containing a high proportion of sucrose or a polyhydric alcohol or alcohols (containing more than one hydroxyl group). Elixirs may also contain ethanol, which means that the majority of these products are considered less suitable for prescribing. An example is Chloral Elixir, Paediatric BP, used for the short-term treatment of insomnia in children.
- **A linctus** is a viscous liquid used to treat cough. Linctuses contain a high proportion of sucrose, other sugars or a suitable polyhydric alcohol or alcohols. To have a full soothing effect on a cough, a linctus should be sipped and swallowed slowly, and must not be diluted. An example of a commonly dispensed linctus is Simple Linctus BP, used for the symptomatic relief of dry tickly coughs.
- **A mixture** describes a pharmaceutical oral solution or suspension, for example Magnesium Trisilicate Mixture BP (which is used to relieve the symptoms of indigestion and heartburn).
- **Oral drops** are oral solutions (or suspensions) that are to be administered in small volumes, using a suitable measuring device, often called a 'dropper'. For example, Cipramil® oral drops are used to treat depressive illness and panic attacks.
- **Syrups** are aqueous solutions that contain sugar. An example of a syrup is Tenormin Syrup, a beta-blocking drug that is used to treat hypertension, angina and arrhythmias.

Oral suspensions

A suspension contains one or more active ingredients suspended in a suitable vehicle. The suspended particles will often settle on standing, but can usually be redispersed easily by shaking (e.g. Trimethoprim suspension, an antibiotic).

Oral emulsions

Oral emulsions are oil-in-water dispersions, and one or more active ingredients are dissolved in one or both phases of the dispersion. Emulsions are a useful formulation in which to present water-insoluble or unpalatable drugs, as the taste can be masked with a more pleasant tasting flavouring (Lund, 1994).

Liquids for other pharmaceutical uses

Liquids are also formulated for topical application for use in body cavities such as the nose, mouth or ears, or on the surface of the skin. Examples include nasal drops, mouthwashes, ear drops, soaks, lotions, paints, tinctures and liniments. Liquid formulations can be administered rectally, as an enema.

Topical semisolids

Topical semisolids are designed to have a local therapeutic effect at the site of application to the skin or mucous membranes. They come in several pharmaceutical formulations, described below.

Creams

A cream is a viscous semisolid, which can be either an oil-in-water emulsion (aqueous cream) or water-in-oil emulsion (oily cream). They are used to deliver drug on to the skin, allowing the drug to be delivered very closely or directly to the required site of action.

Ointments

As well as delivering a drug to the skin, ointments have the added benefit of being more effective emollients than creams (i.e. softening or soothing the skin) because they tend to be more greasy. This is because they generally contain a higher quantity of oil-based products than creams. Because ointments are greasy, they often contain a surfactant (a substance that reduces the surface tension of the product) allowing them to be washed off more easily. Ointments are often used for delivery of medication to deeper layers of the skin, such as the dermis or subcutaneous layer, as ointments cause hydration of the skin, increasing the permeability of the skin to drug molecules.

Gels

Gels are usually aqueous in nature and are used as lubricants, for example to lubricate the probe of an ultrasound machine, or to deliver a drug to the surface or deeper layers of the skin.

Pastes

A paste is a semisolid vehicle with a large concentration of solid material added. Pastes are therefore relatively thick, so they do not spread easily, which can result in localised drug delivery; this has advantages in that the drug is not delivered to healthy areas of the skin. For example, Magnesium Sulphate Paste BP used as a 'drawing' poultice for boils can be irritant when applied to healthy skin.

The practice of extemporaneous preparation

'The pestle and mortar days of preparing medicines have been overtaken by pharmaceutical industrial technology . . .' (Roberts, 1988). This gloomy statement reflects the current position of compounding or extemporaneous preparation in community pharmacy, but not in hospital pharmacy. Whereas the traditional image of extemporaneous preparation conjures up images of creams and unguents mixed patiently by hand (adding ingredients and ensuring thorough mixing, before careful packing into coloured jars and bottles for presentation to the patient with an enigmatic label of 'The Ointment'),

extemporaneous preparation is a thriving activity in hospital pharmacies. For example, many patients receiving intravenous chemotherapy for cancer treatment have a 'custom-made cocktail' of medication prepared for them on an individual basis by specially qualified pharmacy staff. Chapter 4 outlines the roles of members of the pharmacy team involved in such preparation. Patients receiving parenteral nutrition may have deficiencies of particular essential nutrients that can be added to the infusion bags, which are prepared on a daily basis.

This section of Chapter 13 introduces the equipment used in small-scale extemporaneous preparation and the techniques used in the manufacture of medications, and outlines some of the challenges facing pharmacists involved in this area of pharmacy practice.

Compounding equipment

This section outlines the five principal items of equipment required for extemporaneous preparation:

- balances – for weighing ingredients
- measuring cylinders – for accurate checking of volumes of liquid ingredients
- mortar and pestle – for reducing particle size of solid ingredients, and for mixing emulsions
- ceramic or glass slab and palette knife or spatula – for thorough mixing of creams and ointments
- heat sources – to melt solid ingredients for incorporation into other solid ingredients.

Balances

Originally, balances used in dispensing consisted of Class B balances (Figure 13.1), which are still used today in the majority of community pharmacies for weighing powders and other solids in the range 10–100 g. Quantities larger than this are more commonly weighed on a top-pan balance (also known as a Class II balance) (Figure 13.2). Newer balances, such as these top-pan balances, must be calibrated in metric units and marked with maximum and minimum weights that can be measured accurately.

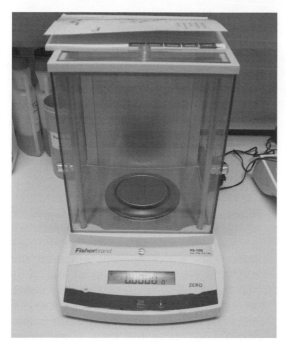

Figure 13.1   A Class B balance used for weighing small quantities of powders.

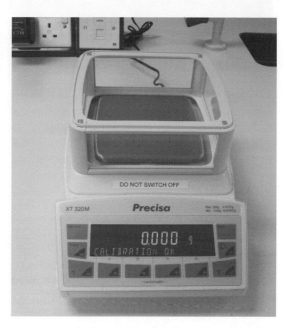

Figure 13.3   A Class I balance used to measure less than 10 grams of an ingredient.

Quantities of less than 10 g should only be measured using a Class I balance (Figure 13.3), although these are rarely found in a community pharmacy setting.

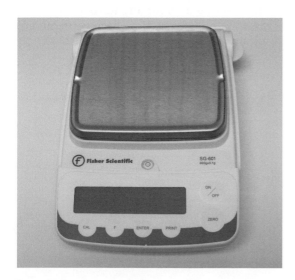

Figure 13.2   A top-pan balance used for measuring more than 10 grams of an ingredient.

Measuring cylinders

Conical measures (Figure 13.4) are used to dispense liquids, although they can be less accurate than cylindrical measures if not used appropriately. This is because cylindrical measures have regular graduations, marked in individual millilitre measurements, whilst conical measures often have uneven divisions in their graduations (Figure 13.4). It is important to understand the correct measuring technique in order to ensure that the correct volume of liquid is dispensed. The level of the liquid should be read from the bottom of the meniscus (see Figure 13.5) with the measure placed on a flat horizontal surface, and with the eye level parallel to that of the liquid's surface.

When pouring the liquid into the dispensing bottle, the cylinder should be allowed to drain thoroughly. Significant quantities of the liquid may adhere to the sides of the measure (especially if the liquid is viscous) and can therefore be lost in transfer. Where possible, only use a single cylinder or conical measure to dispense a liquid, as this significantly reduces error margins

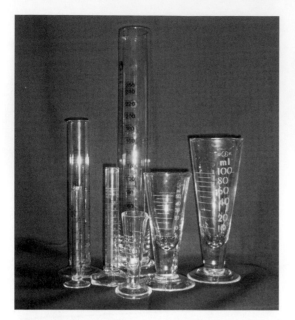

Figure 13.4 A selection of measuring cylinders and conical measures.

– liquids will adhere to the inner surface of a measure, so using more than one measure increases the volume of liquid that will not be dispensed.

Always select the smallest measure possible to contain the required volume of liquid as this also reduces error margins. The use of a large cylinder to measure a small volume of liquid increases the surface area that the liquid must travel across before it reaches the dispensing bottle, increasing the potential for the liquid to adhere to the inner surface. In the case of measuring highly viscous liquids (e.g. glycerol), it is a good idea to measure an excess of the liquid required, and then pour off the volume required into a dispensing bottle, leaving just the excess volume in the measuring cylinder. Don't forget to allow the liquid time to drain back down the sides of the measure to ensure that the correct volume has been dispensed.

Two rules of good practice should be observed when measuring liquids.

- When pouring from a stock bottle, hold the label away from the edge from which you are pouring. This will ensure that the label is not damaged or spoiled by liquids that may run down the outside of the bottle (see Figure 13.6). In the event that a label becomes damaged or hard to read, the label should be replaced immediately. This ensures that anyone using the stock bottle knows what it contains, and the expiry date and batch numbers of the product.
- Hold the cap of the stock bottle in your hand whilst pouring out the required volume. This practice ensures that you put the right cap back on the right bottle, particularly as you may be using more than one liquid. If the wrong cap is put back on a bottle, the bottle must not be used for any further dispensing, as the contents may have been contaminated by any liquids on the inner surface of the cap.

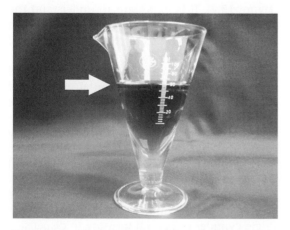

Figure 13.5 The volume is read from the bottom of the meniscus.

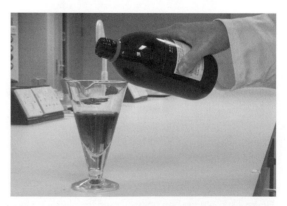

Figure 13.6 Correct pouring technique: protecting the label from spillage or drips.

All measures for liquids used in dispensing procedures must comply with the Weights and Measures Regulations (OPSI, 1994) and be stamped as such.

Mortar and pestle

Historically, the piece of equipment most commonly associated with the pharmacist is the mortar (bowl) and pestle (pounding device) (Figure 13.7), used to reduce the size of solid particles, mix powders, mix powders with liquids and prepare emulsions. Two types are currently available.

- **Glass mortar and pestle combinations** are small and are only suitable for size reduction of crystalline materials, given their smooth surface and low friction. They are ideal for preparations that contain dyes or that stain (e.g. iodine) as the surface does not become discoloured by absorption of the material.
- **Porcelain (or composition) mortar and pestle combinations** are normally much larger than the glass versions and have a rougher surface. They can be used for size reduction, mixing solids and liquids and preparing suspensions and emulsions.

Different sorts of mortar and pestle are available, and it is important to select a 'matching pair'. Some mortars are flat bottomed, whilst others are rounded. The ends of pestles can be flattened or rounded. In order to get the greatest size reduction with the least effort, a flat mortar should be used with a flat pestle. Rounded combinations are more effective for combining solids with liquids.

The correct method of combining the ingredients should also be considered.

- If two small quantities of roughly the same size are to be combined, the ingredients can be added to a suitably sized mortar and mixed well.
- If a small quantity of powder is to be added to a larger quantity of a second ingredient, the process of 'doubling up' is used, to ensure even dispersion of the ingredients. To do this, the smaller quantity is put in the mortar first. Approximately three times as much of the second ingredient is then added and the two mixed carefully using the pestle. Once these two ingredients have been sufficiently well combined, a further quantity of the second ingredient is added (roughly the same volume as that already in the mortar). This should then be mixed carefully using the pestle. This process should be repeated until all the larger quantity has been added.

Box 13.2 provides some hints and tips on working with powders.

Slab and palette knife/spatula

The slab (which may be glass or ceramic) and palette knife or spatula (Figure 13.8) are used

---

Box 13.2   Hints and tips for working with powders

- If powdered ingredients have become clumped or gritty, sieve before use with a 180 μm sieve.
- Powders containing a lot of moisture (e.g. starch) should be dried carefully to improve mixing properties.
- If combining a coloured material into a pale base, break down the coloured material carefully first using a mortar and pestle, otherwise the product may appear speckled.
- Whilst 'doubling up', make sure there is two or three times the volume of base to powder to avoid 'crumbling' of the final product.

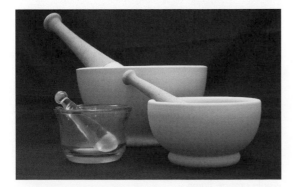

Figure 13.7   A selection of mortars and pestles.

when combining semisolids into a single preparation, in a process known as trituration, used, for example, in the preparation of an ointment. In this process, powders that have been finely ground in a mortar and pestle can be combined with a cream or ointment base (e.g. menthol in aqueous cream, used for the relief of itching from allergic reactions or chickenpox). The powdered crystals and the cream base are placed on the slab and combined using the doubling up procedure described above (see Mortar and pestle). The powdered crystals are rubbed in using the palette knife to ensure even distribution throughout the cream. This process continues until all the crystals have been added. Once the mixing process has been completed, the cream can be smoothed out into a very thin layer so that any large particles can be easily

seen and the mixing process resumed until no solid particles are visible to the naked eye (Figure 13.9).

Heat sources

It is rare in today's pharmacies for a pharmacist to need a heat source to produce an extemporaneous product. In the event that such a product is prescribed for a patient, the pharmacist would normally order it from a 'specials' manufacturer. (A list of special-order manufacturers is provided at the back of the *British National Formulary*.) This section provides a brief overview of heat sources used during the preparation of extemporaneous preparations, as you may be expected to make such products during your undergraduate training. Box 13.3 provides some hints and tips on heating.

An excess quantity of the product required for dispensing should be made, as some material will inevitably be lost during transfer into the dispensing container – a 10% excess of the product should allow for this problem.

- **Bunsen burners** (Figure 13.10) are used to melt small amounts of solids (e.g. menthol crystals) directly in a test tube, or to heat a small water bath mounted on a tripod. For most extemporaneous preparations, a cool flame is sufficient to melt the solid, so the fierce blue flame is not required. When not in

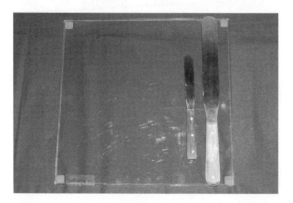

Figure 13.8 Glass slab and palette knives used for trituration.

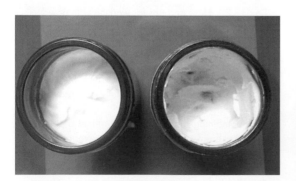

Figure 13.9 A well combined cream (left) – all the ingredients are combined homogeneously, creating a smooth cream – and a poorly combined cream (right) – note the splitting (separation) of the constituents.

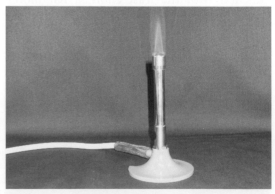

Figure 13.10 A Bunsen burner. In the 'on' position it has a blue flame and in the 'standby' position it has a highly visible orange flame.

use, the Bunsen burner should be turned off, or set to the orange or pilot flame so that it can easily be seen.

- **Water baths** (Figure 13.11) are used when melting large quantities of solids, usually in the preparation of creams and ointments. The ingredients to be melted are usually placed in a porcelain basin and placed in the water at a temperature of 60–80°C to avoid risk of scalding.
- **Electric hot plates** (Figure 13.12) have the advantage that it is easy to control the temperature. In addition, many electric hot plates have a built-in magnetic stirrer so the addition of a 'magnetic flea' allows for constant stirring if two or more solids have to be incorporated into the product.

Box 13.3   Hints and tips on heating

- When melting ingredients to make a cream, ensure all ingredients are heated to about the same temperature before combining.
- Mix slowly and carefully during cooling, to avoid incorporation of air into the product, which will show up as air bubbles in your 'set' product.
- If a product is cooled too rapidly, materials of different melting points will separate out, giving your final product a granular appearance.

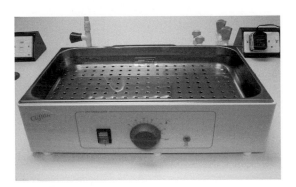

Figure 13.11   A water bath used for melting large quantities of solid ingredients.

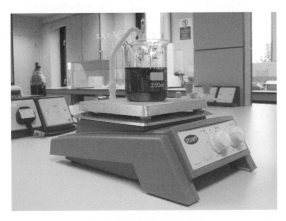

Figure 13.12   An electric hot plate with magnetic flea (stirrer), which allows for constant gentle stirring.

Dispensing extemporaneous preparations

This chapter outlines the methods and procedures that you will use during your degree course, and defines forms of extemporaneous preparation that are commonly seen in pharmacies today. You are encouraged to learn and use these techniques, even though they are not used often in today's community pharmacy setting. The discipline and accuracy developed in this exciting part of your undergraduate studies can be applied to many other parts of the everyday practice carried out in pharmacy. *Pharmaceutical Compounding and Dispensing* (Marriot *et al.*, 2006) is a comprehensive text on extemporaneous preparation and covers in great detail other factors that should be considered by a pharmacist involved in extemporaneous preparation of medications.

References

Lund W (1994). *The Pharmaceutical Codex*, 12th edn. London: Pharmaceutical Press.

Marriot J, Wilson K, Langley C, Belcher D (2006) *Pharmaceutical Compounding and Dispensing*. London: Pharmaceutical Press.

Oxford University Press (2005). *Compact Oxford English Dictionary of Current English*, 3rd edn. Oxford: Oxford University Press.

Roberts D (1988). Dispensing by the community pharmacist: an unstoppable decline? *J R Coll Gen Pract* 38: 563–564.

Royal Pharmaceutical Society of Great Britain (2007). *Medicines, Ethics and Practice: A Guide for Pharmacists and Pharmacy Technicians,* 31st edn. London: Royal Pharmaceutical Society of Great Britain.

OPSI (1994). *Statutory Instrument 1994 No. 1258. The Weights and Measures (Packaged Goods) (Amendment) Regulation.* London: Stationery Office. Available at: www.opsi.gov.uk/SI/si1994/Uksi_19941258_en_1.htm

Winfield A J, Richards R M E, eds (2004). *Pharmaceutical Practice,* 3rd edn. Oxford: Churchill Livingstone.

14

Compliance, adherence and concordance

Rachel L Howard

Introduction

Medicines are one of the most frequently used interventions in UK health care, and their use is increasing every year. In 2006, 752 million prescription items were dispensed in England alone (The Information Centre, 2006a), which is equivalent to every person in England collecting 14 prescription items in a year (The Information Centre, 2006b). This is an increase of 40% since 1995, when an average of 10 prescription items per person were dispensed in England. The majority of these medicines were dispensed to older patients: equivalent to 38 prescriptions per person aged 60 years or over in 2005, nearly double the number dispensed in 1995.

Medicines represent a significant cost to the National Health Service (NHS); £10.3 billion was spent on medicines in 2005, equivalent to £200 per person (The Information Centre, 2007). Over three-quarters of this cost is for medicines dispensed in primary care; 90% of prescriptions were dispensed free of charge to patients.

Although medicines are one of the most frequently used interventions in the developed world, about half of patients do not take their medicines as prescribed, regardless of the condition they are prescribed for, or how long the patient is expected to live (Conrad, 1985; Vermeire *et al.*, 2001; WHO, 2003; Haynes *et al.*, 2005). It is thought that in the developing world even fewer patients take their medicines as prescribed.

Many patients who do not take their medicines will continue to collect their prescriptions from the pharmacy, representing an enormous cost burden to the NHS. Not only do these medicines have to be paid for by the NHS, but medicines that are not taken as prescribed may not work as intended (therapeutic failure) and the patient is less likely to gain benefit. This has been clearly demonstrated in a study exploring the use of immunosuppressant medicines taken to stop the body from rejecting transplanted kidneys. Rovelli *et al.* (1989) found that 18% of patients with a kidney transplant did not take their medicines as prescribed, resulting in either rejection of the transplanted kidney or death in nine out of ten of these patients.

For centuries, the medical profession has been aware that patients do not always do as they are told. Even Hippocrates (who lived in the 5th century BC) was aware that patients sometimes pretended to take their medicines. A number of different terms have been used to describe the behaviour of patients who do not take their medicine as prescribed, including non-compliant and non-adherent. This chapter describes these terms in detail, and introduces the concept of concordance and why it is important. It goes on to consider why patients do not adhere to their medication, and what the consequences of poor adherence might be, and suggests some strategies that can help improve patient adherence, and ways in which pharmacists can use concordance in their daily practice.

What is compliance?

The term compliance has been defined as, 'the extent to which a person's behaviour (taking medications, following a recommended diet or executing lifestyle changes) coincides with medical or health advice' (Kyngas *et al.*, 2000). Until recently patients who did not follow their doctor's instructions were described as 'non-compliant'. However, this term has been criticised because of its negative connotations. 'It suggests yielding, complaisance and submission . . . Non-compliance is a failure or refusal to comply and can imply disobedience' (Vermeire *et al.*, 2001). Use of the term non-compliance also suggests that health professionals have the right to authority over the patient's behaviour (Kyngas *et al.*, 2000). This means that patients have no right to participate in decisions about their health or the medicines they take. By describing patients as non-compliant, we are saying that we expect patients to follow the prescribers' orders unquestioningly. If patients do not, then they may be viewed by health professionals as being irrational and deviant; this contrasts with the patient's perspective of making a rational decision based on their own understanding of

their condition, the treatment, their lifestyle and how they will be affected (Conrad, 1985). This attitude held by health professionals suggests that patients do not have the right to make their own decisions about how they and their bodies will be treated; it is increasingly recognised that this is not appropriate.

The term non-compliance also assumes that prescribed medicines are always beneficial to patients, which is not always the case. Adverse reactions to medicines are the cause of about 5% of admissions to hospital (Pirmohamed *et al.*, 2004); two-thirds of which could be avoided by better management of medicines (Winterstein *et al.*, 2002). Sometimes the alterations patients make to a prescribed regimen can be desirable. For example, Wynne and Long (1996) found that patients who had a stomach bleed whilst taking non-steroidal anti-inflammatory drugs (NSAIDS, e.g. ibuprofen) were more likely to have continued taking their medicine at the dose prescribed than those who did not – those patients who chose to reduce the dose were less likely to experience a serious adverse drug reaction (ADR).

The Royal Pharmaceutical Society of Great Britain (RPSGB, 1997) has described the traditional approach to medicine taking implied by compliance (from a medical perspective) as follows:

> The patient presents with a significant medical *problem* for which there is a potentially helpful treatment. What the doctor or other health professional brings to the situation – scientific evidence and technical expertise – is classed as the *solution*. What the patient brings – 'health beliefs' based on qualities such as culture, personality, family tradition and experience – is classed by clinicians as the *impediment* to the solution. The only sensible way out of this difficulty would appear to be to bring the patient's response to the doctor's diagnosis and proposed treatment, as far as possible into line with what medical science suggests.

Unfortunately, since patients have been non-compliant with medicines for centuries, this approach is unlikely to work. As a result, there has been a gradual shift in thinking in the world of health care. One of these shifts has been to replace the term compliance with adherence.

What is adherence?

The term adherence was introduced in an attempt to reduce the amount of power attributed to health professionals in their relationships with patients (Vermeire *et al.*, 2001). Adherence implies that health professionals have a responsibility to form a 'therapeutic relationship' with patients, in order to encourage them to agree to a recommended treatment regimen. This means that patients should be better informed about their medicines and, in theory, have greater power to decline treatment. This is reflected in the World Health Organization (WHO, 2003) definition of adherence (see Box 14.1). The wording of this definition is similar to the definition for compliance except for two important differences: the definition of adherence:

- incorporates 'agreed recommendations' as opposed to 'medical or health advice'
- recognises the relationship between patients and all health professionals in patient care, not just doctors, by referring to 'healthcare providers'.

The terms 'non-adherence' and 'poor adherence' still refer to patients who do not take their medicine according to the prescribed regimen but are intended to be less judgemental than non-compliance. However, poor adherence still implies that health professionals hold greater power than patients over making decisions that could affect patients' lives (Kyngas *et al.*, 2000).

In the 1990s a working party convened by the RPSGB explored the literature and current expertise on medicine taking (RPSGB, 1997). The working party recommended a shift in perspective away from a compliance/adherence model of medicine taking to 'concordance', which is described in more detail below.

What is concordance?

Concordance was intended to introduce a 'distinct change in culture [and] . . . in teaching about the relationship between prescribing and medicine taking, between patient and prescriber' instead of a 'more politically acceptable way of talking about a technically and morally complex problem' (RPSGB, 1997). Concordance describes the relationship between health professionals and patients. Instead of patients either submitting (compliance) or agreeing (adherence) to decisions made by health professionals, in a concordant relationship the patient is an *equal partner* with the health professional in decision making. This brings greater responsibility for patients and health professionals – patients must begin to take greater responsibility for the consequences of their treatment decisions; health professionals must take greater responsibility for the quality of diagnosis, treatment and explanation (RPSGB, 1997). It must be remembered, however, that not all patients will want greater involvement in decisions about their treatment. In a concordant consultation this preference should be identified – and respected – by the health professional.

In concordant consultations, patients and health professionals contribute different types of expertise and knowledge, which help them to select the most appropriate treatment option. Patients have the opportunity to describe their own (lay) health beliefs and how they experience their condition, and health professionals must enable them to do this. Health professionals

---

Box 14.1   Definitions of compliance and adherence

Compliance

The extent to which a person's behaviour (taking medications, following a recommended diet or executing lifestyle changes) coincides with medical or health advice (Kyngas *et al.*, 2000).

Adherence

The extent to which a person's behaviour – taking medication, following a diet, and/or executing lifestyle changes, corresponds with agreed recommendations from a healthcare provider (WHO, 2003).

must describe their (professionally informed) health beliefs, and the patient should consider these. At the end of a concordant consultation, the patient and health professional will agree a treatment regimen that is acceptable to both parties. This may mean that the patient chooses not to accept the treatment regimen that the health professional believes to be best clinical practice. This differs from a compliance or adherence model in which the patient would make this decision after leaving the consultation (often with inadequate information) and without informing the health professional. Within a concordant consultation the treatment decision is made with the health professional's knowledge and documented in the patient's medical record. This allows future discussion about this decision, more appropriate monitoring of the condition being treated, and an outcome that is acceptable to the patient. If a patient chooses a treatment regimen that the health professional believes will be harmful to the patient, it is still the health professional's right to refuse to prescribe or supply this medicine.

Concordant consultations are challenging for patients and health professionals because they require a dramatic change in the roles and responsibilities of each party. Patients must learn to be open with health professionals, interpret evidence for treatment options, and make decisions about their treatment. Health professionals must learn to be non-judgemental, to help patients be open, to communicate evidence for treatments in non-technical language, and to accept that patients can have the final decision on treatment regimens. Health professionals may be concerned that concordant consultations will take longer than traditional consultations (most consultations in general practice only last 10 minutes) although there is some evidence that health professionals experienced in conducting concordant consultations need not use more time than in a traditional consultation (Dowell et al., 2002).

Finally, because concordance describes the interactions and agreement between patients and health professionals, patients cannot be described as non-concordant, only consultations can be non-concordant.

Why is concordance important?

Misunderstandings can occur if patients and health professionals do not communicate openly. In traditional consultations, health professionals choose the information given to patients about treatment decisions, and patients choose which information about their use of medicines and symptoms they give to health professionals. This minimal communication has led to many misunderstandings (see Box 14.2) (Britten et al., 2000). These misunderstandings can result in patients taking medicines inappropriately, symptoms of ADRs being missed,

---

Box 14.2   Examples of misunderstandings that can occur when patients and health professionals are not open with each other (Britten et al., 2000)

- Patient information not known to the health professional – doctor or pharmacist unaware that patient takes less medication than prescribed
- Health professional information unknown to patient – patient unaware they should reduce the dose of medication they take
- Patient receives conflicting information – patient given different advice by general practitioner and pharmacist
- Disagreement about cause of symptoms – doctor or pharmacist does not accept that symptoms are caused by a medicine, because they believe the computer record (which erroneously says the medicine was first prescribed 2 days earlier) rather than the patient (who correctly says the medicine has been taken for over 2 weeks)
- Failure to communicate health professional's decision: patient misunderstands the diagnosis and therefore cannot understand why the medicine has been prescribed
- Relationship factors: patient continues to take a medicine because they believe the doctor wants them to, whilst the doctor continues to prescribe the medicine because they believe stopping it will upset the patient

conditions being managed suboptimally and patients' anxieties about their illness remaining unresolved. For example, Pollock (2001) describes a lady with gastro-oesophageal reflux disease (a relatively common condition in which stomach acid is regurgitated into the oesophagus, causing heartburn) whose anxieties about the possible causes of her condition are not identified by her doctor. This resulted in her feeling dissatisfied with her treatment and worried about her future, even though her symptoms are well controlled.

Good communication between patients and health professionals about medicines can improve (Stevenson *et al.*, 2004):

- satisfaction with care
- knowledge of the condition and treatment
- adherence to medication or lifestyle changes
- health outcomes
- fewer medication-related problems.

Why do people not adhere to prescribed medicine regimens?

As a health professional, it is easy to feel frustrated when patients do not take their medicines as prescribed. Understanding *why* patients don't take their medicines can help to avoid some of this frustration and, in some cases, enable health professionals to improve patient adherence. A great deal of research has been undertaken to explore why patients don't adhere to their medicines, and more than 200 different reasons have been studied since 1975 (Vermeire *et al.*, 2001). Despite this, however, no single factor can reliably predict whether or not a patient will adhere to their medicine, highlighting the complexity of patients' decisions about medicine taking.

Different types of poor adherence have been divided into a number of categories, which are briefly described in Box 14.3. Although these categories can help us to understand the different ways in which patients are non-adherent, they do little to help us understand why patients do not take their medicines. For

this, we need to dig a little deeper. The WHO (2003) has identified five dimensions of factors thought to influence patient adherence (see Box 14.4), these are described in more detail below.

Social and economic factors

Social and economic factors include age, social class, level of education, employment status, income, level of literacy, lack of effective social support networks, unstable living conditions, and family dysfunction. Many of these factors have been found to impact on patient adherence, although they do not consistently predict which patients will be poorly adherent to medication.

Box 14.3 Categories of non-adherence

Primary vs secondary

- Primary non-adherence: patient does not have prescription for medicine dispensed
- Secondary non-adherence: patient has medicine dispensed but does not take it according to the prescribed regimen

Intentional vs unintentional non-adherence

- Intentional non-adherence: patient chooses not to take their medicine according to the prescribed regimen
- Unintentional non-adherence: patient either forgets, or is unable, to take their medicine according to the prescribed regimen

---

Box 14.4 Five dimensions of adherence (WHO, 2003)

- Social/economic factors
- Health system/healthcare team factors
- Condition-related factors
- Therapy-related factors
- Patient-related factors

Age

Age is associated with different levels of adherence. Poor adherence to medicines is higher in adolescents and elderly patients (but still present in all age groups). In adolescents this could reflect rebellion against the control that a medication regimen can impose on their lives. In elderly patients this can be due to the complexity of medication regimens and presence of multiple disease states.

Poverty

Poverty can have an impact on patients' ability to pay for prescriptions. Within the NHS, prescriptions are provided free of charge for patients on low incomes, which should lessen the impact of poverty on adherence. In other healthcare systems (such as the USA), however, inability to pay for prescriptions continues to be a problem (Wamala *et al.*, 2007).

Ethnic origin

Ethnic origin has also been found to influence adherence, and this has been linked to cultural beliefs about medicines and causes of disease, and levels of trust in the medical profession.

Healthcare team and system-related factors

As suggested in the section on concordance, good relationships and communication between patients and health professionals are important in helping patients to adhere to their medication (Conrad, 1985; Vermeire *et al.*, 2001). Haynes *et al.* (2005) suggest that maintaining contact between patients and health professionals is likely to be the most important factor in helping patients adhere to medication. Brookhart *et al.* (2007) support this view: they found that patients were 3–6 times more likely to restart statin therapy (medicine used to lower cholesterol levels) following an appointment with a doctor.

Conversely, healthcare systems with poorly trained or overworked health professionals, short consultation times, inadequate patient education and follow-up, and lack of help for patients to pay for treatment can contribute to poor adherence.

Condition-related factors

Many conditions and diseases create demands on patients that affect their ability or desire to adhere to their medicines. Patients with particularly severe symptoms or rapidly progressing disease may be more likely to adhere to agreed treatment regimens, whilst patients with depression are often less likely to be adherent to medication. This can be particularly important in patients with other conditions such as heart disease and diabetes who are also likely to have depression.

Therapy-related factors

The medicines prescribed can also influence patients' ability or desire to adhere. Complex regimens are associated with poor adherence. Medication regimens can be complex because they contain multiple different medicines, or because they need to be taken several times a day. Levels of adherence decrease as the number of times a medication should be taken each day increases. Although there is not much difference between levels of adherence between once and twice daily regimens (75% and 69% of all doses are taken, respectively), adherence is much lower with regimens that require medication to be taken three or four times daily (65% and 51% of all doses taken, respectively) (Claxton *et al.*, 2001). Adverse effects from medicines are infrequently cited as a cause of poor adherence (Vermeire *et al.*, 2001).

Patient-related factors

Patient-related factors include patients' knowledge and beliefs about, and attitudes to, medicines and disease. Patients' beliefs are increasingly thought to be the most important factor influencing adherence (RPSGB, 1997;

Box 14.5   Types of patients' beliefs about medicines
(RPSGB, 1997)

- Perceived efficacy of medicine
- Danger of becoming immune over time
- Unnaturalness of manufactured medicines
- Danger of addiction and dependence
- Anti-drug attitude
- Balancing risks and benefits

Horne & Weinman, 1999; Vermeire *et al.*, 2001)
(see Box 14.5 and detailed descriptions below).
Often, patients' beliefs contribute to poor
adherence because they are not recognised by
health professionals. This can cause a breakdown in communication and misunderstandings between patients and health professionals
(RPSGB, 1997).

Perceived efficacy

Patients' beliefs about whether their medicine
will work are particularly important. This perception will not just affect a patient's initial decision of whether or not to take a medicine; it will
also be reviewed at regular intervals whilst they
are taking their medicine. Patients may decide
whether or not to continue taking their medicine on the basis of how well their symptoms are
controlled. In some cases, this may seem relatively straightforward. For instance, if a patient
has pain that is then relieved by painkillers, it
might seem obvious to a health professional
that the patient should continue to take the
medicine. However, some patients who take
painkillers for a long time and no longer experience pain may wonder if they need the
painkillers any more, and may therefore 'test'
the efficacy of their painkillers by stopping them
and seeing if the pain returns. If the pain does
not return, then they will stop taking the
painkillers. If the pain does return, however, it
can sometimes take a number of days for the
patient to regain adequate pain control.
    Testing the efficacy of a painkiller is relatively
simple for a patient to do. It is more difficult,
however, for patients to assess the efficacy of an

antihypertensive. Hypertension is rarely associated with symptoms (although patients often
associate it with headaches). If a patient believes
that they can tell when their blood pressure is
raised, and only takes their medication when
they believe they are experiencing symptoms,
then they may stop taking the medication. This
may seem inappropriate from a health professional's perspective.

Immunity over time

Patients may believe that they will become
immune to the effects of a medicine if they take
it for prolonged periods of time. This may be
related to government messages about over-
prescribing of antibiotics leading to increased
bacterial resistance (RPSGB, 1997); however,
patients can hold the belief that they will
develop immunity to many different types of
medicine. This belief leads some patients to take
'holidays' from their medicines, leading to deterioration in disease control which in some cases
can be dangerous. For instance, if a patient
suddenly stops taking their beta-blocker, reflex
tachycardia (a fast heart rate) may result, exacer-
bating a patient's angina pain. Not only can
patients experience symptoms from their illness
(sometimes warranting hospital admission), but
when they do start taking their medication
again, it can be more difficult to regain control
of their symptoms.

Unnaturalness of manufactured medicines

Patients may believe that Western medicines,
many of which are manufactured from synthetic
compounds, are 'unnatural'. In this sense, some
patients may perceive such medicines to be
unhealthy and therefore avoid taking them. In
contrast, non-Western medicines such as herbal
remedies are considered to be natural and therefore less likely to be harmful. Patients who
believe this can be reluctant to take Western
medicines prescribed by their doctor.

Danger of addiction and dependence

Some patients perceive themselves to have
become dependent on their medicines (Conrad,

1985), and they may therefore feel that they have lost control of their lives. Some patients will alter their medicine regimen in order to help regain some control. This has been particularly noted in chronic diseases such as epilepsy. In addition, patients fear that they may become addicted to their medicine. This includes medicines for which addiction is not thought to be pharmacologically plausible. For example, many patients believe that they can become addicted to selective serotonin reuptake inhibitors (SSRIs, e.g. paroxetine) used to treat depression because they experience adverse effects if they stop taking them suddenly. In some cases, these adverse effects can make it difficult for a patient to stop taking SSRIs. However, SSRIs do not induce addiction in the pharmacological sense. Patients prescribed medicines, such as SSRIs, that can precipitate adverse effects if stopped suddenly should be counselled about the hazards of stopping their medicine suddenly.

Anti-drug attitude

Many patients perceive the word drug negatively because of an association with illicit drugs. Illicit (or recreational) drugs such as amphetamines, cocaine and opioids are frequently associated with a risk of physical, mental and moral harm (RPSGB, 1997). This perception can be transferred to medicines used for therapeutic reasons, creating a fear of taking 'drugs', or being perceived as a 'drug user'. Referring to prescribed drugs as medicines is unlikely to overcome this stigma, but is preferable to calling them drugs.

Managing everyday life

Everyday life can make it difficult for some patients to follow their doctor's instructions. For example, Bissell *et al.* (2004) describe how an Asian patient struggled to follow the diet dictated to her by health professionals to help control her type 2 diabetes because she had to cook separate meals for herself and the rest of her family. Patients may also experience difficulties incorporating their medicines into a busy daily routine, particularly if medicines need to be taken more than twice a day. Adjustments to

medicine regimens are perhaps best illustrated by patients who take diuretics to help control fluid retention in congestive cardiac failure. These patients experience a diuresis (increased urine flow) which can make it difficult to be far from a toilet. Many of these patients will alter the timing of their diuretic if they need to go shopping. This alteration is rarely discussed with health professionals, although the majority of health professionals would recommend that patients amend their regimen in this way.

Alternatively, some patients may use drugs such as tranquillisers to control the symptoms of everyday life, particularly during stressful events such as divorce or bereavement.

Non-acceptance and stigma of illness

Admitting that they have an illness can impact on a patient's sense of identity, and some patients may be unwilling to accept that they are unwell. This can be a particular problem when the treatment for the illness is perceived to be obvious to others, for example inhaler therapy for asthma or injecting insulin for diabetes. In addition, some illnesses are perceived to be heavily stigmatised. For instance the seizures that characterise primary generalised epilepsy (which used to be called grand mal epilepsy) have been considered to be signs of demonic possession (Jilek-Aall, 1999). Other illnesses in which the patient is in some way perceived to be at fault, such as HIV/AIDS can also be heavily stigmatised. Hence, some patients can be reluctant to admit they have a stigmatised illness. Where patients do not accept that they have an illness, they are significantly less likely to take the prescribed medicine (Horne & Weinman, 1999).

Balancing risks and benefits

Most patients who take medicines will have a view about the risks of taking medicines generally, or the specific medicine they have been prescribed. This view will be based on various sources of information, including relatives, friends, the media, the internet and health professionals. Patients will usually make a risk–benefit assessment on the basis of their understanding about the risks of taking the medicine against the perceived benefits. Patients may include the following in their risk assessment:

* possibility of experiencing adverse effects (and their severity)
* effect on lifestyle and quality of life
* taste, smell, size and shape of medicines.

Patients may not make their risk–benefit analysis immediately; instead they may choose to 'trial' the medicine and assess the impact of adverse effects on their lifestyle. From a health professional's perspective, this can be particularly problematic when patients are likely to experience short-term adverse effects such as flatulence with statins, or drowsiness and nausea with opioid analgesics. Warning patients that they may experience short-term adverse effects (and when they are likely to resolve) may help to prevent patients from deciding that the risks of medicine taking outweigh the benefits. Horne and Weinman (1999) found that patients who perceived the risks of a medicine to outweigh the potential benefits were significantly less likely to be adherent to the prescribed regimen.

Communication between doctors and patients about medicines may affect patients' risk–benefit analysis. In particular, focusing more on the adverse effects of medicines, rather than the benefits, may encourage patients to choose not to take them. The information contained in patient information leaflets (PILs) has been criticised for having a greater focus on the risks (adverse effects) of medicines than on the benefits. As a result, PILs are being changed to redress this balance (Connelly, 2005). Less is known, however, about whether communication between health professionals and patients is changing.

What are the consequences of poor adherence to medication?

In general, patients who are poorly adherent to their prescribed medicine regimens have poorer outcomes than patients who are considered to have good adherence. Table 14.1 shows the outcomes of poor adherence to medication for a variety of conditions. In most of these studies, poor adherence is defined as taking less than 75–80% of the prescribed doses, although some studies define poor adherence as taking less than 100% of doses (Simpson *et al.*, 2006).

How can adherence to medication be improved?

Despite our better understanding of the causes of poor adherence to medication regimens, finding ways to help patients take their medicines as prescribed remains a challenge. Strategies to improve patient adherence differ depending on whether a patient is prescribed short-term therapy (such as a course of antibiotics) or long-term therapy (Haynes *et al.*, 2005).

Counselling patients and giving them written information about their medication have proved effective. Phone calls to remind patients to take their medicines have also been shown to help, for example, telephone reminders after 3 days of treatment with *Helicobacter pylori* eradication therapy have improved patient adherence (Haynes *et al.*, 2005). (*H. pylori* is a bacterium associated with an increased risk of peptic/gastric ulcers.)

Strategies to improve adherence to long-term therapy have limited efficacy. Even the most effective strategies offer only small improvements in medication use and health outcomes. In general, successful strategies to improve medication adherence with long-term therapy involve multiple interventions:

* more convenient care
* increased information
* reminders to take medication
* self-monitoring of effectiveness (such as blood pressure)
* psychological therapy
* telephone follow-up.

Examples of some successful interventions are shown in Table 14.2 and are discussed in more detail below.

Table 14.1 Consequences of poor adherence to prescribed medicine regimens

Reference	Reason for medication	How adherence was assessed	Consequences of poor adherence
Vik *et al.*, 2004	Multiple conditions	Unknown	8–11% of hospital admissions in older patients were attributed to poor adherence to medication
Simpson *et al.*, 2006	Multiple conditions comparing active and placebo medication	Unknown	Patients with poor adherence to active or placebo medication were twice as likely to die as patients with good adherence
Kimmel *et al.*, 2007	Anticoagulation	Percentage of bottle openings compared with prescribed frequency	Poorly adherent patients (those with 20% fewer or 10% more bottle openings than prescribed) were more than twice as likely to have a subtherapeutic INR, and nearly twice as likely to have a supratherapeutic INR
Hope *et al.*, 2004	Congestive cardiac failure	Percentage of prescribed doses collected from pharmacy and percentage of bottle openings compared with prescribedf requency	Poor adherence was associated with more frequent emergency hospital visits for cardiovascular disease
Ho *et al.*, 2006a	Diabetes mellitus	Percentage of prescribed doses collected from pharmacy	Poorly adherent patients were 1.6 times more likely to be hospitalised and 1.8 times more likely to die than patients with good adherence (defined as those who collected > 80% of their prescriptions)
Nachega *et al.*, 2007	HIV	Percentage of prescribed doses collected from pharmacy	Poor adherence to medication was associated with fewer patients achieving suppression of HIV load. With each 10% increase in prescription collection above 50%, an additional 10% of patients achieve viral load suppression
Ho *et al.*, 2006b	Post-MI	Percentage of prescribed doses collected from pharmacy	Patients who stopped taking aspirin, beta-blockers or statins after an MI were nearly 4 times more likely to die than patients who continued treatment.
Rasmussen *et al.*, 2007	Post-MI	Percentage of prescribed doses collected from pharmacy	Patients with poor adherence to beta-blockers or statins were 25% more likely to die than patients with good adherence No difference was found in mortality between patients with good or poor adherence to calcium channel blockers.

INR, international normalised ratio, a measure of blood clotting; MI, myocardial infarction

Table 14.2 Examples of interventions that have improved patient adherence

Patient group	Successful interventions	Reference
Patients with tuberculosis	Pharmacist education about medication	Clark *et al.*, 2007
Multiple patient groups	Medication reminder packaging	Heneghan *et al.*, 2006
Patients with hypertension or hyperlipidaemia	Dispensing medicines in blister pack; pharmacist-led education about medicines; regular follow-up with a pharmacist	Lee *et al.*, 2006
Multiple patient groups	Motivational interviewing	Rubak, 2005
Patients with HIV/AIDS	Improving practical medication management skills with individual patients over at least 12 weeks	Rueda *et al.*, 2006
Patients with hyperlipidaemia	Simplified medication regimens; improved patient information and education; reminders	Schedlbauer *et al.*, 2004
Patients with hypertension	Simplifying dosage regimens; medicine reminder charts; social support and family support	Schroeder *et al.*, 2004

Patient education

Educating patients about their medicines is unlikely to be effective on its own (Schroeder *et al.*, 2004; Haynes *et al.*, 2005) although it has been successful in some patient groups (Clark *et al.*, 2007). Indeed, the traditional model of a pharmacist counselling about medication (without assessing patients' existing knowledge or desire for information) has been found to alienate patients (Salter *et al.*, 2007). This does not mean that educating patients about their medicine is not important, but it needs to be combined with an attempt to elicit what patients want from their treatment, how their beliefs will affect their medication taking, their current level of understanding, and to help patients decide whether or not to take the recommended medication (RPSGB, 1997).

Multicompartment compliance aids

Multicompartment compliance aids (MCAs) (also known as monitored dosage systems (MDSs)) such as dossett boxes, NOMAD systems

and Medidos, are generally considered to be overused (Nunney and Raynor, 2001). Patients using them often think they would remember their medicines without them, and some have difficulties opening the medicine compartments. This may be because patients are rarely asked which MCA they would prefer (often pharmacies only keep one type of MCA). In addition, using MCAs reduces patients' knowledge about the medicines they take. However, MCAs do help patients in some groups to remember their medicines and are likely to be beneficial.

Regular contact with health professionals

Haynes *et al.* (2005) argue that maintaining contact between health professionals and patients is likely to be the most effective strategy to improve adherence to medication. This view is supported by Brookhart *et al.* (2007), who found that patients who had stopped taking their medication after a myocardial infarction were most likely to start taking it again if they had had recent contact with a doctor, and particularly if this was with the prescribing doctor.

Is improving adherence to medication always beneficial to patients?

Health professionals assume that improving patient adherence to medication will be beneficial to patients, but this may not always be true. In some cases, increased adherence may have no impact on clinical outcomes, whilst in others it may lead to more adverse effects. For example:

- a pharmacy care programme improved patient adherence to statins, but did not improve lipid control (Lee *et al.*, 2006)
- directly observed therapy for tuberculosis (where patients take three-times weekly doses of medication under health professional observation) and standard therapy (where patients take daily therapy at home) showed no differences in terms of course completion or clearance of tuberculosis infection (Volmink & Garner, 2006)
- patients with gastrointestinal bleeding associated with NSAIDs are more likely to have taken the prescribed dose of NSAID than patients without gastrointestinal bleeding (Wynne & Long, 1996)
- good adherence in clinical trials to medication that was subsequently found to be harmful tripled the risk of death (Simpson *et al.*, 2006).

Simpson *et al.* (2006) also found that patients with poor adherence to placebo and active medication were both twice as likely to die as patients who had good adherence. This suggests that the positive benefit of good adherence to medication is likely to be due to good overall healthy behaviour. Rasmussen *et al.* (2007), however, found that patients with good adherence to beta-blockers and statins (both known to reduce mortality after a myocardial infarction) had better outcomes than patients with good adherence to calcium channel blockers (medicines for which there is no evidence that they reduce mortality risk after a myocardial infarction). This study suggests that good adherence to effective and safe medication is beneficial irrespective of other health behaviours.

What does concordance mean, in practice, for pharmacists?

So far this chapter has described the different meanings of compliance, adherence and concordance, why patients do not adhere to prescribed regimens and the potential consequences of this. In addition, it has introduced some of the interventions that may help patients adhere to their medication. But what does concordance mean, in practice, for pharmacists?

It is clear from multiple studies that the traditional approach to medicine taking, which expects patients to adhere to the prescribed medication regimen, is ineffective. Pharmacists therefore need to adopt a more concordant approach to their interactions with patients. At first glance, it may be difficult to see how the traditional pharmacist role lends itself to concordant consultations. However, every time a pharmacist interacts with a patient they have an opportunity for a concordant consultation. Some of these opportunities, and how they can be used, are described below.

Dispensing medication

When pharmacists dispense medication for patients, they are ideally placed to identify any practical problems that patients might experience with their medicines. Such practical problems could include not knowing when or how to take their medication, and inability to open medicine containers or to read labels. Pharmacists can ask patients about these issues when dispensing medicines for the first time, and also when patients present with a repeat prescription. In addition, patients' understanding of information provided by the doctor can be checked. This can provide patients with an opportunity to ask their pharmacist questions about medicine efficacy or side-effects. When answering such questions, it is important to identify what the patient has been told by the doctor, to avoid giving conflicting information. Pharmacists can also take the opportunity to talk to patients about their expectations for the medicine and their perspective on whether or not to take the medicine.

Repeat dispensing

Pharmacists are increasingly involved in repeat dispensing systems. In this case, the pharmacist may be the only contact the patient has with a health professional for up to 6 months. It is therefore important that the pharmacist asks simple questions such as, 'How are you getting on with your medicines?', to help identify any practical problems the patient may be experiencing, or symptoms that could be adverse effects of the medication. In addition, pharmacists can use this opportunity to discuss with the patient whether they are taking the medication as prescribed; if not, why not; and if the level of non-adherence is likely to pose a risk to the patient.

Medicine use reviews

Under the new Pharmacy Contract, pharmacists can provide medicines use reviews (see Box 6.7). These provide an ideal opportunity to sit down with a patient in private and talk with them about their medicines as part of a concordant consultation. This allows pharmacists to identify any problems that a patient is experiencing, talk to them about their understanding of their medicines and why they take (or do not take) them.

Prescribing

Pharmacists can now qualify as supplementary or independent prescribers (see Chapter 2), which provides an ideal opportunity for a concordant consultation. Pharmacists can discuss patients' health beliefs, and the benefits and risks of the available treatment options, in order to agree with patients their preferred treatment strategy. This can also include anticipating (and resolving) practical problems with treatment, such as administering medication several times a day.

Taking medication histories when patients are admitted to hospital

Hospital pharmacists are increasingly involved in making accurate records of what medications a patient who is admitted to hospital has been taking at home. This is an ideal time for a concordant consultation, which can help to inform how the patient is treated throughout their admission. Pharmacists can identify whether patients take their medicine as prescribed, why they may choose to alter the prescribed regimen, what practical difficulties they may experience, and their beliefs about their medicines. This information can then be used to help doctors agree suitable treatment regimens with patients during the admission, and on discharge from hospital.

Counselling patients about medicines on discharge from hospital

Hospital pharmacists are often involved in medication counselling before patients are discharged home. This provides an opportunity to discuss patients' beliefs and understanding about their medicines and conditions, their intention to take the medication, and any practical difficulties they may anticipate when they return home.

Developing a concordant approach

Pharmacists need to develop new skills in order to have concordant consultations with patients (Weiss, 2004). The skills required at each stage of a concordant consultation are described in Box 14.6. In addition, pharmacists must carefully examine their attitudes to patients and the impact these attitudes could have on a consultation. It is important that pharmacists care for, respect and trust the patient (Weiss, 2004). Pharmacists should also be aware of their own values, beliefs, history, needs and culture, and how these can influence interactions with different patients. This awareness should allow

Box 14.6 Pharmacists' skills for a concordant approach

Greet the patient

- Greet the patient appropriately and introduce yourself as the pharmacist
- Ensure the patient's comfort and privacy
- Reassure the patient so that they feel you have time for them; treat them as an equal partner
- Identify barriers to communication, such as deafness or language barriers
- Establish how involved the patient wants to be in decision making
- Set boundaries for the discussion, such as subjects you can discuss and how much time is available
- Be alert to the patient's reactions and tailor your approach to each individual (try not to scare them)

Explore the patient's issues

- Identify why the patient has come to see you
- Elicit the patient's view of their illness, their psychosocial and emotional issues
- Discuss their expectations

Question the patient

- Use open questions, and avoid leading questions, wherever possible (see Chapter 8, page 78)

Actively listen to the patient

- Give the patient your full attention
- Do not interrupt them
- Respond to verbal and non-verbal cues (see Chapter 8, page 78)

Empathise with and support the patient

- Acknowledge the patient's views and concerns in a non-judgemental fashion, using appropriate non-verbal cues such as nodding, leaning forward and open posture to encourage patients to speak
- Ask probing questions to elicit further responses
- Discuss the patient's concerns and views, and encourage them (and allow them time) to ask you questions

Clarify and summarise the patient's responses

- Check your understanding of what the patient has said (and show you have been listening) by summarising your understanding

Know your limitations

- Ensure that your knowledge is up-to-date
- Avoid discussing topics you do not understand (refer the patient to someone else if necessary)

Share information with the patient

- Offer to share your thinking on the problem
- Explain why examinations are needed
- Discuss the benefits and risks of the treatment options with the patient in language they can understand (avoid jargon)
- Check that the patient has understood what you have said

Agree the issues with the patient

- Elicit the patient's reaction to, and feelings about, the information given
- Negotiate a treatment plan that is acceptable to both you and the patient
- Identify (and resolve) any practical difficulties the patient may experience in adhering to the treatment

Finish the consultation and plan for the future

- Summarise the decision that has been reached
- Explore whether the patient has anything else to discuss (offer an additional consultation if necessary)
- Agree with the patient what happens next (when/if they come back to see you, what they do if there is a problem)
- Communicate the outcome of the consultation to other relevant health professionals (with the patient's agreement)

(Weiss, 2004; Clyne et al., 2007)

pharmacists to adapt their communication style to individual patients' needs.

Summary

This chapter has shown that taking medicines is a complex issue, influenced by many factors. How patients take their medicines can have positive and negative impacts on both their health and their relationships with health professionals. Health professionals' approach to patients' medicine-taking behaviour is changing, illustrated by the change in terminology from compliance, through adherence, to concordance. Concordance remains a challenging model of care for patients and professionals, with as-yet uncertain benefits. Pharmacists can engage in concordant consultations in most aspects of their work, but for pharmacists to be truly concordant in their approach to patients they will need to learn new skills and reflect on their attitudes to their patients.

References

Bissell P, May C R, Noyce P R (2004). From compliance to concordance: barriers to accomplishing a re-framed model of health care interactions. *Soc Sci Med* 58: 851–862.

Britten N, Stevenson F A, Barry C A, *et al.* (2000). Misunderstandings in prescribing decisions in general practice: qualitative study. *BMJ* 320: 484–488.

Brookhart M A, Patrick A R, Schneeweiss S, *et al.* (2007). Physician follow-up and provider continuity are associated with long-term medication adherence: a study of the dynamics of statin use. *Arch Intern Med* 167: 847–852.

Clark P M, Karagoz T, Apikoglu-Rabus S, *et al.* (2007). Effect of pharmacist-led patient education on adherence to tuberculosis treatment. *Am J Health Syst Pharm* 64: 497–505.

Claxton A J, Cramer J, Pierce C (2001). A systematic review of the associations between dose regimens and medication compliance. *Clin Ther* 23: 1296–1310.

Clyne W, Granby T, Picton C (2007). *A competency framework for shared decision-making with patients. Achieving concordance for taking medicines.* Keele, National Prescribing Centre Plus. www.npc.co.uk/ pdf/Concordant_Competency_Framework_2007.pdf.

Connelly D (2005). User testing of PILs now mandatory. *Pharm J* 275: 12.

Conrad P (1985). The meaning of medications: another look at compliance. *Soc Sci Med* 20: 29–37.

Dowell J, Jones A, Snadden D (2002). Exploring medication use to seek concordance with 'non-adherent' patients: a qualitative study. *Br J Gen Pract* 52: 24–32.

Haynes R B, Yao X, Degani A, *et al.* (2005) Interventions to enhance medication adherence. *Cochrane Database Syst Rev* issue 4, CD000011.

Heneghan C J, Glasziou P, Perera R (2006). Reminder packaging for improving adherence to self-administered long-term medications. *Cochrane Database Syst Rev* issue 1, CD005025.

Ho P M, Rumsfeld J S, Masoudi F A, *et al.* (2006a). Effect of medication nonadherence on hospitalisation and mortality among patients with diabetes mellitus. *Arch Intern Med* 166: 1836–1841.

Ho P M, Spertus J A, Masoudi F A, *et al.* (2006b). Impact of medication therapy discontinuation on mortality after myocardial infarction. *Arch Intern Med* 166: 1842–1847.

Hope C J, Tu W, Young J, *et al.* (2004). Association of medication adherence, knowledge, and skills with emergency department visits by adults 50 years or older with congestive heart failure. *Am J Health Syst Pharm* 61: 2043–2049.

Horne R, Weinman J (1999). Patients' beliefs about prescribed medicines and their role in adherence to treatment in chronic physical illness. *J Psychosom Res* 47: 555–567.

Jilek-Aall L (1999). Morbus sacer in Africa: some religious aspects of epilepsy in traditional cultures. *Epilepsia* 40: 382–386.

Kimmel S E, Chen Z, Price M, *et al.* (2007). The influence of patient adherence on anticoagulation control with warfarin: results from the International Normalized Ratio Adherence and Genetics (IN-RANGE) Study. *Arch Intern Med* 167: 229–235.

Kyngas H A, Duffy M E, Kroll T (2000). Conceptual analysis of compliance. *J Clin Nurs* 9: 5–12.

Lee J K, Grace K A, Taylor A J (2006). Effect of a pharmacy care program on medication adherence and persistence, blood pressure, and low-density lipoprotein cholesterol: a randomized controlled trial. *J Am Med Assoc* 296: 2563–2571.

Nachega J B, Hislop M, Dowdy D W, *et al.* (2007). Adherence to nonnucleoside reverse transcriptase inhibitor-based HIV therapy and virologic outcomes. *Ann Intern Med* 146: 564–573.

Nunney J M, Raynor D K T (2001). How are multi-compartment compliance aids used in primary care? *Pharm J* 267: 784–789.

Pirmohamed M, James S, Meakin S *et al.* (2004). Adverse drug reactions as cause of admission to hospital: prospective analysis of 18 820 patients. *BMJ* 329:15–19.

Pollock K (2001). "I've not asked him, you see, and he's not said": understanding lay explanatory models of illness is a prerequisite for concordant consultations. *Int J Pharm Pract* 9: 105–117.

Rasmussen J N, Chong A, Alter D A (2007). Relationship between adherence to evidence-based pharmacotherapy and long-term mortality after acute myocardial infarction. *J Am Med Assoc* 297: 177–186.

Rovelli M, Palmeri D, Vossler E, *et al.* (1989). Noncompliance in organ transplant recipients. *Transplant Proc* 21: 833–834.

Royal Pharmaceutical Society of Great Britain (1997). *From compliance to concordance, achieving shared goals in medicine taking.* London: Royal Pharmaceutical Society of Great Britain.

Rubak S (2005). Motivational interviewing: a systematic review and meta-analysis. *Br J Gen Pract* 55: 305–312.

Rueda S, Park-Wyllie L Y, Bayoumi A M, *et al.* (2006). Patient support and education for promoting adherence to highly active antiretroviral therapy for HIV/AIDS. *Cochrane Database Syst Rev* issue 3, CD001442.

Salter C, Holland R, Harvey I, *et al.* (2007). "I haven't even phoned my doctor yet." The advice giving role of the pharmacist during consultations for medication review with patients aged 80 or more: qualitative discourse analysis. *BMJ* 334: 1101–1104.

Schedlbauer A, Schroeder K, Peters T J, *et al.* (2004). Interventions to improve adherence to lipid lowering medication. *Cochrane Database Syst Rev* issue 4, CD004371.

Schroeder K, Fahey T, Ebrahim S (2004). Interventions for improving adherence to treatment in patients with high blood pressure in ambulatory settings. *Cochrane Database Syst Rev* issue 3, CD004804.

Simpson S H, Eurich D T, Majumdar S R, *et al.* (2006). A meta-analysis of the association between adherence to drug therapy and mortality. *BMJ* 333: 15–18.

Stevenson F A, Cox K, Britten N, *et al.* (2004). A systematic review of the research on communication between patients and health care professionals about medicines: the consequences for concordance. *Health Expect* 7: 235–245.

The Information Centre (2006a). *Report of hospital prescribing, 2005.* www.ic.nhs.uk/statistics-and-data-collections/primary-care/prescribing/report-of-hospital-prescribing-2005 (accessed 25 April 2007).

The Information Centre (2006b). *Prescriptions dispensed, 2005.* www.ic.nhs.uk/statistics-and-data-collections/primary-care/prescribing/prescriptions-dispensed-2005 (accessed 25 April 2007).

The Information Centre (2007). *Prescription cost analysis, 2006.* www.ic.nhs.uk/statistics-and-data-collections/primary-care/prescriptions/prescription-cost-analysis-2006 (accessed 25 April 2007).

Vermeire E, Hearnshaw H, Van Royen P, *et al.* (2001). Patient adherence to treatment: three decades of research. A comprehensive review. *J Clin Pharm Ther* 26: 331–342.

Vik S A, Maxwell C J, Hogan D B (2004). Measurement, correlates, and health outcomes of medication adherence among seniors. *Ann Pharmacother* 38: 303–312.

Volmink J, Garner P (2006). Directly observed therapy for treating tuberculosis. *Cochrane Database Systematic Rev,* issue 2, CD003343.

Wamala S, Merlo J, Bostrom G, *et al.* (2007). Socioeconomic disadvantage and primary non-adherence with medication in Sweden. *Int J Qual Health Care* 19: 134–140.

Weiss M (2004). Educational perspectives on concordance. In: Bond, C, ed. *Concordance.* London: Pharmaceutical Press.

Winterstein A G, Sauer B C, Hepler C D, *et al.* (2002). Preventable drug-related hospital admissions. *Ann Pharmacother* 36: 1238–1248.

WHO (2003). *Adherence to long-term therapies. Evidence for action.* Geneva: World Health Organization.

Wynne H A, Long A (1996). Patient awareness of the adverse effects of non-steroidal anti-inflammatory drugs (NSAIDs). *Br J Clin Pharmacol* 42: 253–256.

15

Sale and supply of medicines: risk and advice provision

Rachel L Howard

Introduction

The sale and supply of medicines is an important part of the pharmacist's role. It is also one of the most potentially dangerous roles that pharmacists undertake. It is therefore important for pharmacists to be aware of:

- the potential risks associated with medicines
- how the sale and supply of medicines is controlled to minimise these risks
- the roles and responsibilities of pharmacists when selling or supplying medicines.

The sale and supply of medicines has many sources of risk for pharmacists, pharmacy employees and customers; examples are shown in Box 15.1. In addition, there are risks associated with the services that pharmacists provide, such as supplying prescriptions, selling medicines over the counter (OTC), and counselling patients about medicines or other public health issues. If these services are not delivered to the highest standards, there is a risk of harm to members of the public. In addition, there is also a risk of financial loss to pharmacists through compensation claims from injured patients, lost earnings because of suspension from work, and loss of business. Pharmacists who do not provide pharmacy services to a high enough standard also risk being removed from the Pharmaceutical Register. Many factors will affect the ability of a pharmacist to deliver these services to the highest standards, some of which are described in Box 15.2.

Box 15.1 Examples of sources of risk in a community pharmacy

- **People:** customers and staff members may carry infections or be aggressive
- **Equipment:** lifting heavy objects, or lifting inappropriately, risks injury
- **Materials:** pharmacies may contain a number of hazardous materials in addition to medications, including compressed gases
- **Building design:** fire precautions must be taken into account

---

Box 15.2   Factors that affect a pharmacist's ability to deliver services

- Dispensary design – cramped conditions impair the flow of dispensing work and increase the risk of dispensing errors
- Availability of a well-equipped private counselling area to ensure customer privacy and confidentiality
- Good systems of communication between members of staff in the pharmacy, and with prescribers, nurses, patients and carers
- Reporting systems to record near misses, dispensing errors, interventions on prescriptions and advice given to customers if felt appropriate
- Skill mix – ensuring appropriate members of staff are on duty to allow work to flow smoothly and safely
- Leadership: the pharmacy will run more smoothly and safely if well managed

---

This chapter concentrates on managing the risks associated with the sale and supply of medicines. A detailed discussion of other risks that may impact on pharmacy businesses is available in Butler (2005). In this chapter we introduce the legal and ethical considerations relevant to the sale and supply of medicines, risk management, how to respond if an error reaches a patient and what constitutes negligence.

Legal and ethical considerations when selling and supplying medicines

This section presents a brief overview of the legal and ethical considerations relevant to the sale and supply of medicines. More detailed descriptions can be found in the *Medicines, Ethics and Practice Guide for Pharmacists and Pharmacy Technicians* (MEP) and *Dale and Appelbe's Pharmacy Law and Ethics* (Appelbe & Wingfield, 2005a).

Legal considerations

The sale and supply of medicines and other substances offered for sale by registered pharmacies is controlled by a wide variety of laws, acts and regulations that implement Europe-wide directives and regulations within England, Scotland and Wales (although the implementation of these recommendations differs slightly across the UK). These include the Medicines Act 1968, Misuse of Drugs Act 1971, and the Medicines for Human Use Regulations 2005, which control the manufacture, labelling, distribution, sale and supply of medicines. Although the dates on some of these acts and regulations may seem old, they are updated regularly through amendments. For example, the regulations governing the sale and supply of controlled drugs have undergone dramatic changes in recent years following the Shipman Inquiry. (More information can be obtained from www.the-shipman-inquiry.org.uk.) It is therefore essential for pharmacists to maintain up-to-date knowledge of the laws, acts and regulations that influence their practice. An overview of how these laws, acts and regulations influence the sale and supply of medicines is given in Table 15.1.

Licensed products (marketing authorisations)

Wherever possible, pharmacists should supply licensed medicinal products to the public. These are products that have been granted a marketing authorisation (MA) (formerly known as a product licence). This guarantees the safety, quality and efficacy of the medicine. An MA is granted when a manufacturer submits the necessary paperwork confirming the safety, quality and efficacy of the medicine to either the Medicines and Healthcare products Regulatory Agency (MHRA) in the UK, or the European Medicines Evaluation

Table 15.1   A selection of laws and regulations that affect the practice of pharmacy and the sale and supply of medicines by pharmacists

Law, act or regulation	What the law, act or regulation means for pharmacists supplying medicines
European Community Council Directives and Regulations (enacted in the UK through the acts and regulations listed below)	Dictates the procedures for authorisation and supervision of medicinal products for human and veterinary use. Includes: • requirements for a marketing authorisation • good manufacturing practice for human and veterinary medicines • standards and protocols for tests on medicines for human use • requirements for medication advertising, labelling and leaflets; wholesale distribution of medicines; colouring agents that can be added to medicines; manufacture, sale and supply of controlled drugs; data protection
Medicines Act 1968 (and its subsequent amendments)	Applies to all medicines for human use (when they are being used as medicines); defines three classes of medicines for human use: • general Sales List (GSL): available for sale without a pharmacist's supervision • pharmacy medicines (P): only available for sale from a registered pharmacy under the supervision of a pharmacist (GSL medicines purchased from a registered pharmacy can only be sold when a pharmacist is on the premises) • prescription-only medicines (POM): only available for supply in response to a prescription written by an authorised prescriber Also imposes controls on the sale and supply of herbal and homoeopathic remedies (Appelbe & Wingfield, 2005a).
Veterinary Regulations 2005 Poisons Act 1972	Replaces the Medicines Act 1968 for medicines for veterinary use Controls the sale of non-medicinal poisons. A list of non-medicinal poisons is published in the MEP. Poisons are listed in two parts. • Poisons in Part I and Part II can be sold by a person lawfully conducting a retail pharmacy business. • Poisons in Part II can also be sold by a listed seller (a person whose name is entered on a local authority list). Also defines seven schedules that impose different restrictions on the sale of non-medicinal poisons. Schedules 1 and 4 are most relevant to pharmacies: • Schedule 1: Details special restrictions on storage, sale and record keeping. • Schedule 4: Details products that are exempt from controls under the Poisons Act.
Chemical (Hazard Information and Packaging for Supply) Regulations 1994 (CHIP)	CHIP controls the classification, packaging and labelling of substances that are dangerous to supply (except medicinal products and those covered by the Medicines Act 1968). Where these are stored in a pharmacy, CHIP regulations must be adhered to.
Control of Substances Hazardous to Health Regulations 1999 (COSHH)	Under COSHH regulations, employers must assess the risk of chemicals which employees are exposed to in the workplace, and limit those risks through the implementation of appropriate procedures, which employees must follow.
Medicines for Human Use Regulations 2005	Controls the sale and supply of medicines by ensuring all products have a marketing authorisation (except for products exempt under Schedule 1, which can be supplied on a named-patient basis (unlicensed medicines), and setting guidelines for the wording of labelling (Schedule 3) and patient information leaflets (Schedule 4). Schedule 2 sets out the penalties for failure to comply with these regulations.

Table 15.1   Continued

Law, act or regulation	What the law, act or regulation means for pharmacists supplying medicines
Misuse of Drugs Act 1971	Classifies controlled drugs into five schedules with different levels of control applied to them: • Schedule 1 (CD Lic) • Schedule 2 (CD POM) • Schedule 3 (CD No Register) • Schedule 4 Part I (CD Benz) • Schedule 4 Part II (CD Anab) • Schedule 5 (CD Inv) Changes have been made to the Misuse of Drugs Act in response to the Shipman Inquiry and extension of prescribing rights to supplementary and independent non-medical prescribers. Details of the restrictions on controlled drugs are available in the MEP.
Alcoholic Liquor Duties Act 1979	Controls the manufacture, sale and supply of denatured alcohol. Both methylated spirits and isopropyl alcohol can be supplied by pharmacists. Sale and supply of these denatured alcohols is controlled by this act.
Denatured Alcohol Regulations 2005	Sets out the requirements for manufacture, supply, receipt, sale, and storage of all forms of denatured alcohol.
Civil and statutory (criminal) law	Includes the Medicines, Poisons and Misuse of Drugs Acts because transgressing from these acts may result in prosecution.

MEP, *Medicines, Ethics and Practice Guide for Pharmacists and Pharmacy Technicians* published by the Royal Pharmaceutical Society of Great Britain.

Agency (EMEA) in Europe. If insufficient evidence is supplied, a MA will not be granted.

Medicinal products with a MA can be identified from the MA number, which is printed on the packaging of all authorised medicines (unless the packaging is considered too small to contain all the relevant information). There may, however, be circumstances where a licensed product is not available. In this case, a supply of an unlicensed medicine can be made (see section on supplying unlicensed medicines, page 159).

The MA specifies (amongst other things):

• the product description
• the conditions for which the medicine may be used – the licensed indications
• the dose range for each licensed indication – the licensed doses
• how the packaging should be labelled (see Chapter 12).

It also specifies the need for a patient information leaflet (PIL) and the specific product characteristics (SPC) (also known as the summary of product characteristics), which details licensed indications and doses, cautions and contraindications, drug interactions, mode of action, and pharmacokinetics of the medicine. SPCs and PILs for the majority of licensed medicines are available free of charge via www.medicines.org.uk. Further information on the process for obtaining an MA is available from MHRA (2006a) and the EMEA (2007).

Ethical considerations

In addition to the legal considerations, the sale and supply of medicines is guided by biomedical ethics and the ethical principles of the pharmacy profession, which are described in the MEP. The key ethical responsibilities of the pharmacist are shown in Box 15.3. The code of ethics for pharmacists has recently been amended following consultation with members of the profession and has been published in the *Code of ethics for pharmacists and pharmacy technicians* (RPSGB, 2007), which is is supplemented by the *Professional standards and guidance documents* (available via the RPSGB website (www.rpsgb.org)).

Indemnity insurance

One aspect of the code of ethics that is commonly overlooked by newly qualified pharmacists is the requirement to have adequate personal professional indemnity insurance (RPSGB, 2007). This ensures that the pharmacist is able to pay compensation if a patient is injured as a result of the pharmacist's actions. Before 1991, pharmacists employed by hospitals were exempt from prosecution under statutory law because they had Crown immunity, and many viewed professional indemnity insurance as unnecessary. This is no longer the case, however, as all hospital staff, including pharmacists, can now be prosecuted. Prosecution is rare, but can occur when a pharmacist commits an offence under the Medicines Act. Such an offence can include a dispensing error that reaches the patient.

Some pharmacists wrongly believe themselves to be covered by their employer's indemnity insurance. Under some circumstances the employer may try to recoup the costs of a lawsuit from the employee pharmacist responsible for an injury. Also, the employing pharmacy may not be at fault. In this case, the injured patient may bring a civil case for compensation against the individual pharmacist. *All* pharmacists should therefore ensure they have personal professional indemnity insurance that gives them adequate cover for the type of work they do. Different policies are available depending on the area of pharmacy worked in and the type of work done (such as community, hospital, primary care or locum pharmacists).

Selling over-the-counter medicines

Medicines sold from a pharmacy (as opposed to those supplied in response to a prescription) are collectively described as OTC medicines. There is no formal list of Pharmacy ('P') medicines, or a statutory list of medicines that may be sold from a pharmacy. Instead, any medicines on the general sales list (GSL), and any medicines not included on the prescription-only medicines (POM) list, are eligible for sale from a registered pharmacy. The classification of a medicine can be found in the *British National Formulary* (BNF) or SPC. ('P' medicines will be those not classified as GSL or POM.) In addition, a list of medicinal products classified as GSL, P or POM is available in the MEP.

Pharmacists are also able to sell herbal remedies and food supplements (vitamins and minerals). Although there are some controls under the Medicines Act, the sale of these is largely unregulated. Many patients view herbal remedies and food supplements as harmless alternatives to licensed medicines. Manufacturers of herbal remedies and food supplements often make claims that their products will help a variety of conditions, although these may not necessarily be supported by any evidence. It is important that pharmacists who sell these products are aware of their associated risks. These include potentially toxic ingredients, interactions with licensed medicines such as warfarin, and adverse effects.

Box 15.3 Ethics for pharmacists

'Ethics is the science of morals, or moral philosophy' (Appelbe & Wingfield, 2005a).

The Code of Ethics for pharmacists published by the RPSGB sets out seven key ethical principles that pharmacists should adhere to (RPSGB, 2007):

- Make the care of patients your first concern
- Exercise your professional judgement in the interests of patients and the public
- Show respect for others
- Encourage patients to participate in decisions about their care
- Develop your professional knowledge and competence
- Be honest and trustworthy
- Take responsibility for your working practices.

Box 15.4 Roles and qualifications of pharmacy support staff

Medicines counter assistants

Defined as any assistant who is delegated to sell medicines under a protocol (RPSGB, 2006a). They should have taken, or be undertaking, an accredited course relevant to their duties. Such courses should cover the knowledge and understanding associated with Pharmacy Services S/NVQ Level 2 units entitled; 'assist in the sale of OTC medicines and provide information to customers on symptoms and products; assist in the supply of prescribed items (taking in a prescription and issuing prescribed items)' (RPSGB, 2006a).

Dispensing/pharmacy assistants

These assistants should have completed or be working towards qualifications in:

• sale of OTC medicines and provision of information to customers on symptoms and products
• prescription receipt and collection, assembly of prescribed items (including label generation)

• ordering, receiving and storing pharmaceutical stock
• supply of pharmaceutical stock
• preparation for manufacture of pharmaceutical products (including sterile and non-sterile production).

They should be enrolled on a suitable training programme (e.g. Pharmacy Services S/NVQ Level 2, or an equivalent accredited programme) within 3 months of commencing their role and should complete their training within 3 years.

Pharmacy technicians

Should have successfully completed Pharmacy Services S/NVQ Level 3 (or equivalent qualifications). Once complete, technicians can volunteer to be on the Pharmaceutical Register. (There are plans to make registration of pharmacy technicians compulsory in the future.)

OTC sales of licensed medicines can only be made by a registered pharmacist or an appropriately qualified member of pharmacy support staff (see Box 15.4) under the supervision of a pharmacist. Even GSL products cannot legally be sold from a registered pharmacy unless a pharmacist is in control of the premises; at present this means that a pharmacist must be physically on the premises when a sale is made.

Members of the public sometimes expect all OTC medicines to be completely safe for them to take. It is the pharmacist's job to ensure that the medicine which is sold is appropriate for the purchaser to use, effective and safe (or as safe as is practicable). No medicine is completely safe. Aspirin, for example, can cause gastrointestinal bleeding in an otherwise healthy young person, although the risk is much higher in an older person who has had a stomach bleed in the past. The pharmacist should therefore ensure that customers are aware of how to take their medicine, the risks associated with that medicine,

and what to do if a problem occurs. As part of the sale, the pharmacist should obtain sufficient information from the customer to satisfy themselves that the medicine is safe and appropriate. The RPSGB Practice Committee (2000) has issued guidance on the sale of OTC medicines (also known as counter prescribing). This identifies five stages in the counter-prescribing process:

• recognising and interpreting the condition
• determining the goal of treatment
• recommending a treatment
• providing advice
• recording the intervention (if appropriate).

These stages are described in more detail in Box 15.5.

Pharmacist supervision of OTC sales has increased in importance with a series of 'POM to P switches' in which a medicine that has previously been available only on prescription (POM) is made available through a pharmacy (P). These drugs have been carefully assessed for their

---

Box 15.5   Guidance on counter prescribing

Recognise and interpret the condition

- Find out who the patient is – it may not be the person in front of you.
- Ask what symptoms the patient has, and how long they have had them for.
- Find out what (if any) other medication they are taking (or have taken recently) – could this be causing the symptom, or is this another treatment for the symptoms?
- Ask if the patient has any other symptoms. If the patient is in front of you, look for other signs such as whether or not they look unwell.
- Take particular care if the patient is a baby, infant or child, pregnant or breastfeeding, or elderly. Refer patients who present with potentially serious symptoms, symptoms of long duration, or from a high risk group (if appropriate).

Determine the goal of treatment

- Ask the patient (or their representative) what they want to achieve with the medicine. Do they want to cure, reduce, or eliminate their symptoms; arrest or slow the progression of their condition; prevent a disease or pregnancy?
- Consider whether the patient's goal is achievable with the medicines available from you.

Recommend a treatment

Based on your assessment of the information you have obtained in the previous two stages, you should recommend a treatment for the patient. This could involve:

- giving advice on how to manage the symptoms without a medicine (self-care) and/or reassurance,

without recommending a medicine or other treatment

- recommending a medicine or other treatment
- referring to someone else such as the patient's general practitioner or hospital emergency department, depending on the urgency of the symptoms.

Provide advice

When making a recommendation, the following advice or information should be given to the customer:

- why you have chosen this course of action and how the customer can best achieve the intended outcomes
- what assessment you have made of their condition, any changes that they should monitor for and what to do if they occur
- how to use the recommended treatment
- under what circumstances the customer should seek further advice, and who they should seek advice from.

Record the intervention

In order to allow monitoring of the treatment that has been recommended and allow audit of interventions, a record of the intervention should be made (in appropriate cases) on a patient medication record system. Reflecting on these interventions can also help develop a pharmacist's continuing professional development record.

(RPSGB Practice Committee, 2000)

---

safety to the public, but have the potential to mask more serious conditions if used inappropriately. Examples of POM to P switches include omeprazole (sold OTC to treat heartburn, but could mask stomach cancer if used inappropriately) and simvastatin (a cholesterol-lowering drug available OTC at a dose that has no evidence of benefit; it should not be taken by patients with, or at a high risk of developing, cardiovascular disease).

Supplying prescribed medicines

In addition to being sold OTC, GSL and 'P' medicines can also be supplied in response to a valid prescription signed by an appropriate practitioner such as a doctor, dentist, supplementary or independent prescriber. By contrast, POMs can only be supplied in one of three situations:

- if a valid prescription is issued by an appropriate practitioner
- under a patient group direction (PGD)
- as an emergency supply.

The requirements for a valid prescription are described in Chapters 9 and 10 and in the MEP.

A PGD is a written direction relating to supply and administration (or administration only) of a POM to a patient, signed by a doctor or dentist, and a pharmacist. This allows the supply or administration of a POM to a patient where the conditions specified in the PGD are met.

Pharmacists can make emergency supplies of POM medicines at the request of a patient, doctor or a prescribing nurse or pharmacist (but not a dentist). In order to do this, a pharmacist must be confident that there is a valid reason for the request (such as running out of tablets whilst on holiday or over a bank holiday), and that a valid prescription has been issued to the patient for that medicine in the past. Further information about emergency supplies is available in the MEP.

Patients' expectations for the supply of prescribed medicines

When a patient receives a supply of a prescribed medicine there is a basic level of service that they can expect, governed by the legal and ethical considerations of medication supply. Patients expect medication supplies to be accessible, accurate, prompt, of appropriate quality, of sufficiently long expiry date, and packaged and labelled for the recipient. Each of these expectations is described in more detail below.

- **Accessible:** patients expect the pharmacy to be open at the times advertised. If a pharmacy is not open at these times, there are two consequences: a breach of the contract with the primary care trust (PCT) for dispensing National Health Service (NHS) prescriptions, and loss of revenue because the patient is likely to go elsewhere.
- **Accurate:** medication supplied to the patient should be an accurate reflection of the medication prescribed. Patients do not expect dispensing errors to occur.

- **Prompt:** patients do not expect to wait for long periods of time for their prescriptions. Where there is likely to be a delay in supplying a medicine, the patient should be informed of this (and the reason why). The patient should also be given the opportunity to take their prescription elsewhere if this is the case.
- **Appropriate quality:** patients expect the supplied medicines to be of a quality that is safe for them to take. Therefore, patients should never be supplied with medicines that have been stored inappropriately. For example, if fridge monitoring shows that a medicine stored in the fridge has not been kept at the appropriate temperature (usually 2–8°C), the medicine should not be supplied. In addition, medicines returned from patients' homes should not be reused because the conditions of storage cannot be guaranteed.
- **Sufficiently long expiry date:** patients expect their medicines to be within the expiry date for the duration of the course. If this is not possible, for example if a 14-day course of an antibiotic liquid with a 7-day expiry is prescribed, the patient should be able to collect a further supply to enable them to complete the course.
- **Packaged and labelled for the recipient:** patients expect to be able to identify which medicines are theirs. All dispensed medicines should therefore be individually packaged for that patient, with a label stating only the patient's name, name of the medication and directions stating how to take the medication (also see Chapter 11). Directions should be given in language that patients can understand. This means avoiding legal jargon and complex medical or pharmaceutical terminology or abbreviations. Even simple directions can be misunderstood by patients, so understanding should be checked diplomatically before a patient leaves the pharmacy (Davis *et al.*, 2006).

Service expectations for the supply of prescribed medicines

Simply meeting patients' expectations for the supply of prescribed medicines is not enough. In addition, there are legal and ethical considerations associated with the supply of medicines that patients may be unaware of. These set the minimum standards for supplying prescribed medicines to patients and are described in detail below.

- A prescribed medicine should always be supplied under the supervision of a pharmacist. This means that the pharmacist must have assessed the prescription, either before or after the medicine has been dispensed (but before it is supplied to the patient).
- A pharmacist must make a professional assessment of the prescription. This should encompass whether the prescription is legal (is all the appropriate information on the prescription and is the pharmacist confident that the prescription is not a forgery?) and whether the prescription is appropriate. Judgements regarding the appropriateness of the prescription should be made based on the available information, such as patient age, other medication on the prescription, medication on the patient medication record (PMR), prescription charge exemption (pregnancy, diabetes, etc.), and questioning the patient if appropriate.
- Every pharmacy should have procedures in place to minimise the risk of a dispensing error, or contamination of a medicine with another substance.
- If the prescribed medicine is a product with an MA, then this product should be supplied (rather than a product prepared in the pharmacy or a cheaper product without an MA).
- Prescribed medicines cannot be substituted in a community pharmacy. Thus the specific brand or strength of medicine prescribed should be dispensed. If that brand or strength is not available, it should be ordered in, or the prescriber should be contacted to confirm that an alternative brand or strength can be supplied (and the prescription amended accordingly). (See Chapter 10, page 104, for guidelines on endorsing prescriptions.)
- Child-resistant closures (CRCs) should be used on all medicines, unless a patient specifically requests otherwise. If such a request

is made, it should be documented on the patient's PMR.
- All dispensed medicines should be supplied with clear, legible, indelible labels. Labels should include appropriate additional cautions and warnings. A list of additional warning labels is provided in Appendix 9 of the BNF (see Chapter 11).
- If the full quantity required on a prescription cannot be supplied, the patient should be offered the opportunity to take the prescription elsewhere.
- The dispensed medicines should be supplied direct to the patient or carer wherever possible.

Supplying unlicensed medicines

Under the Medicines for Human Use (Marketing Authorisations, etc.) Regulations 1994, certain medicinal products that do not have an MA can be supplied in response to a valid prescription signed by a doctor, dentist or supplementary prescriber for use by an individually named patient (MHRA, 2006b). When a prescriber issues such a prescription, they take on responsibility for any adverse events resulting from the use of the medicine. (If a medicine has an MA, then the manufacturer will take some responsibility for adverse events resulting from the use of the medicine within its licence.) The pharmacist supplying the unlicensed medicine may also take on some responsibility for adverse events.

When a pharmacist supplies an unlicensed medicine they should consider the following points.

- Is supplying the medicine in the best interest of the patient? This decision should be based on the evidence base for the prescribed medicine; the availability of alternative treatments for the patient's condition; and whether the patient has tried these alternatives.
- A pharmacist can refuse to supply the medicine if the risks to the patient appear to outweigh the potential benefits.

If the pharmacist decides to supply the medicine, they should:

- ensure that the patient is aware the medicine is unlicensed, but without undermining confidence in the medicine or the prescriber
- keep a record for 5 years of the: source of the product; person to whom, and the date on which, the product was sold or supplied; quantity of each supply; batch number of the product supplied; details of any adverse reactions to the product (any serious suspected adverse reactions should be reported to the MHRA via the Yellow Card Scheme (see Chapter 3, page 27), indicating that the product is unlicensed).

Further information on the supply of unlicensed medicines is available from the MHRA (2006b), and the RPSGB (2004).

Preventing errors when selling or supplying medicines

As discussed in Chapter 6, errors are inevitable during the working life of a pharmacist. However, every pharmacist has an ethical responsibility to minimise the risk of errors occurring. Pharmacists can be removed from the Pharmaceutical Register if they repeatedly make errors in the course of their work (this has serious implications for their conscience as well as their financial wellbeing). There is also a legal incentive to minimise errors because pharmacists can be prosecuted if a patient is harmed as a result of a dispensing error or failure to correct a high-risk prescription (see Boxes 15.11–15.14).

Dispensing errors

Dispensing errors are a relatively uncommon – but nevertheless important – area of risk in community pharmacy, with the potential to cause harm to the patient and possibly result in criminal proceedings against the pharmacist. In community pharmacy, at least four incorrect items per 100 000 items dispensed will be handed out to patients (Ashcroft *et al.*, 2005), with a further 22 incorrect items per 100 000 items dispensed identified at the checking stage

(near misses). These figures are likely to underestimate the actual number of near misses and dispensing errors that occur in community pharmacy.

The most common types of dispensing error are:

- selecting the wrong drug, or wrong quantity or strength of drug
- making a mistake on the label
- putting the wrong medicines in a patient's bag.

Pharmacists are more likely than any other member of the pharmacy support staff to make dispensing errors that reach patients because the medicines they dispense often do not receive a second check from another person (Ashcroft *et al.*, 2005). Pharmacy support staff also make a large number of errors that are subsequently identified at the final check. Many factors are associated with an increased risk of dispensing errors; some of which are shown in Box 15.6 (Ashcroft *et al.*, 2005). Although second checking of prescriptions is known to reduce the risk of dispensing errors reaching patients, over a quarter of prescriptions are dispensed by the pharmacist alone, with no second check by another member of staff (Ashcroft *et al.*, 2005). This practice should be avoided wherever possible. To help pharmacists reduce the risk of errors occurring, a framework of practice called clinical governance (described below) has been introduced.

Box 15.6 Factors that may contribute to dispensing errors in community pharmacy

---

- Poor lighting
- Distractions and interruptions
- Look-alike and sound-alike medicines
- Inexperienced staff
- Stress
- High workload or insufficient staff members
- Dispensing large numbers of prescriptions
- Pharmacist fatigue
- Misreading prescriptions
- Selecting the wrong medication from a patient medication record

Clinical governance

Clinical governance is one of the ways in which pharmacists ensure the delivery of a high-quality service to members of the public. It incorporates a number of tools that individual pharmacists and pharmacy employees can use to improve the level of service they provide. When the level of service is improved, the risk of errors occurring is reduced. Further information on clinical governance is available from the RPSGB website (www.rpsgb.org/registrationandsupport/clinicalgovernance) and the MEP. The different processes involved in clinical governance are described below.

Accountability

Pharmacists are accountable for their individual professional practice and the standards of service provision in their pharmacy. They are therefore responsible for ensuring that the dispensing of medicines, policies and procedures, clinical advice given to patients and professionals about treatment, and sale and supply of medicines are performed to such a level that the risk of errors is minimised.

Audit

Audit is defined by the RPSGB as the 'systematic evaluation of professional work against set standards' (MEP). Every community pharmacy must carry out at least two audits annually. The subject of one of these audits will be directed by the local PCT as part of the community Pharmacy Contract; the subject of the second audit can be selected by pharmacy staff to make it relevant to their practice and customer base. Community pharmacies are not limited to conducting two audits a year. The RPSGB has prepared a number of audit templates that pharmacies may wish to undertake, including: the accuracy and completeness of PMRs, the dispensing process, recording of interventions on prescriptions, provision of patient counselling, and prescription waiting times. The templates for these and many other audits are available from www.rpsgb.org/registrationandsupport/audit/index.html.

Clinical effectiveness

For a pharmacist to be able to identify prescribing errors (or high-risk prescriptions) and to be able to provide a safe counter prescribing service, they must be aware of current evidence for treatments and apply this to their practice. Part of the application of this knowledge to their practice should involve monitoring patients' care, including drug interactions and adverse drug reactions. Where a pharmacist judges it to be clinically necessary, they should contact the patient's general practitioner and advise them of any risk to the patient. This contact should be recorded as an intervention on the patient's PMR. Guidance on recording interventions is available from the RPSGB (2006a).

Continuing professional development

One way to ensure clinical effectiveness is to undertake continuing professional development (CPD), defined in the MEP as a 'framework for maintaining professional competence'. CPD involves a cyclical process of learning (see Figure 15.1) which allows you to identify learning needs from day-to-day practice instead of relying on the provision of continuing education.

CPD can be undertaken in a number of different forms, including workshops, distance learning courses, conferences, structured reading, talking to colleagues, everyday practice, staff meetings, professional audits and research projects, preparing teaching for others, and

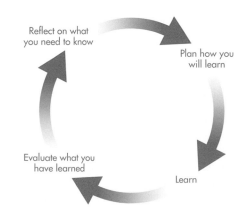

Reflect on what you need to know

Plan how you will learn

Evaluate what you have learned

Learn

Figure 15.1   Learning cycle for CPD.

work shadowing. Individual pharmacists should select the type of learning that suits them best. Pharmacists are advised to record 12 entries over the course of a year in order to comply with the mandatory CPD framework. Further information on CPD is available from the CPD website www.uptodate.org.uk.

Patient and public involvement

Knowing whether the service you provide meets patients' expectations is difficult if you don't ask them. The RPSGB therefore expects pharmacists with an NHS contract to undertake a patient satisfaction survey at least annually. This will help pharmacists to tailor the services they provide to meet the needs of the local population.

Remedying underperformance

Pharmacists should use CPD to ensure that they update themselves on subject areas that they are unsure about. Pharmacists who are not performing to the standards expected by the RPSGB should be identified at a local level and the cause of their substandard performance addressed. Where lapses in standards are short term and do not pose a risk to patients, these

can be dealt with informally. If, however, the lapse is long term (e.g. related to a drug or alcohol problem) then it should be dealt with formally and, if necessary, the pharmacist removed from duties to prevent any risk to patients whilst the problem is addressed. Further information on how underperformance is dealt with is available from the RPSGB (2005b).

Risk management

Risk has been defined in numerous ways, but one of the most simple approaches is to think of risk as, 'the potential for an unwanted outcome' (Butler, 2005). The aim of risk management is to get it right first time, avoiding an unwanted outcome. Risk management is an opportunity to assess whether an unwanted outcome is possible (evaluating the potential risk of it occurring), how likely it is to occur, and how the unwanted outcome can be avoided (developing potential solutions). Pharmacists should ensure that robust risk management procedures are in place. These should include:

- proactively identifying potential risks
- retrospectively recording (see Box 15.7):
  - errors (e.g. where the wrong medicine is given to a patient)

Box 15.7   Near miss and error reporting

All pharmacies should maintain a record of near misses and errors. For this record to be useful, it should be regularly reviewed to identify common trends. This information can then be used to develop new working practices to avoid these near misses and errors in the future. For example, two drugs with similar names may be stored close to each other on the shelves, resulting in frequent dispensing errors. By separating these drugs, or sticking warning labels on the shelves, the number of dispensing errors could be reduced. In some cases (particularly where an error has reached a patient, or where a near miss is particularly common) an in-depth investigation of the cause of the error or near miss will be warranted. This will involve talking to members of staff (and the public) involved in the incident, collating relevant documentation such as standard operating procedures and

dispensing records, and reviewing this evidence to identify possible causes of the error. The ultimate aim of this process, known as root cause analysis, is to amend working practice to avoid a similar error occurring again. This process is time consuming and therefore cannot be applied to all near misses.

Some chains of pharmacies (or independent pharmacies who work closely together) may share their near miss reporting across the group. This allows individual pharmacies to learn from mistakes that have happened elsewhere, further reducing the risk to patients. In addition, some pharmacies may submit their near miss and error reports to the National Reporting and Learning Scheme, which is a national error reporting scheme that receives error reports from all areas of healthcare practice in England.

- near misses (e.g. where the wrong medicine is dispensed, but identified during checking)
- adverse events (e.g. where a patient, member of the public or staff member is injured)
- developing potential solutions, including:
  - standard operating procedures (SOPs) (see Box 15.8)
  - recording interventions made with prescribers (RPSGB, 2006b)
  - developing a procedure for dealing with complaints
  - adequate procedures for checking stock rotation and expiry dates
  - keeping appropriate records of fridge temperatures, which are reviewed regularly and acted on if fridge temperatures are outside the recommended range.

Staff management

Community pharmacists are responsible for managing the staff working in their store(s).

Managers of individual pharmacies are responsible for managing the pharmacy support staff (medicines counter assistants, dispensing/pharmacy assistants and technicians). Managers of chains of stores are also responsible for managing other pharmacists, including locums. Part of a manager's responsibility is to ensure that all staff are appropriately qualified and all staff (including locums) receive an appropriate induction before they start work. Further information on the necessary qualifications for pharmacy support staff can be found in the MEP (also see Box 15.4).

When mistakes are made

It is inevitable that every pharmacist will make a mistake at some point in their career, although with luck and good risk management these mistakes will not result in patient harm. When mistakes do reach patients, however, they are likely to be upset, whether or not they have

---

Box 15.8   Standard operating procedures (SOPs)

SOPs provide a detailed description of the processes to be followed within individual pharmacies. The topics which should be covered, as a minimum, include:

- prescription handling
- assessing the prescription for validity, safety and clinical appropriateness (the clinical or professional check)
- making interventions and problem solving
- assembling and labelling the required medicine or product
- accuracy (or final) checking
- transfer of the medicine or product to the patient.

Individual pharmacists or pharmacy managers may choose to develop additional SOPs for other areas of practice. Pharmacists who delegate tasks to members of the pharmacy support staff must detail within their SOPs the necessary qualifications for an individual to undertake that task.

SOPs should be followed wherever this is practicable, irrespective of whether the pharmacist who

wrote the SOP is present within the pharmacy. SOPs should, however, allow sufficient flexibility to avoid a situation in which staff deliberately do not follow the SOP because it is too onerous. This is best achieved by including staff in the development of SOPs.

Well-written and appropriately used SOPs can help to:

- assure the quality and consistency of the service provided by a pharmacy
- ensure that good practice is achieved at all times
- fully utilise the expertise of all members of the pharmacy team
- enable pharmacists to delegate appropriate tasks, freeing up time for other activities
- clarify who does what in the pharmacy
- provide advice and guidance to locums and part-time staff and train new members of staff.

Guidance on producing SOPs is available from the RPSGB (2001).

been harmed. Sometimes mistakes will be identified by the pharmacy staff, but more often the patient or their relative will identify the error and return to the pharmacy.

When a patient experiences a physical injury as a result of a dispensing error, this is a major threat to trust between the patient and the pharmacist or pharmacy. 'Trust is the cornerstone of the [pharmacist]–patient relationship . . . that trust is sharply challenged when things go wrong' (Leape, 2007). When a patient is harmed by a medication error, there is likely to be an emotional injury in addition to a physical injury, both of which must be treated appropriately to reduce the risk of long-term harm to the patient and their relationship with the pharmacist. But it is not just the patient who will be distressed; relatives and the members of staff involved can also become distressed (Leape, 2007). How pharmacy staff respond to a patient or relative informing them of an error can dramatically impact on the patient's wellbeing, the staff's wellbeing and the likelihood of litigation.

Process for complaints

Patients have a number of different routes by which they can report a dispensing error. Some will come direct to the pharmacy, others to their general practitioner, the PCT, their solicitor or the RPSGB. The RPSGB provides guidance to members of the public on how to make complaints (2005a). Each move up this complaint chain is an escalation in terms of the severity of the complaint and potential impact on career and finances. If a patient or relative brings a complaint direct to the pharmacy it is best to mitigate the risk of an escalation at first contact through good communication.

The RPSGB (2006c) has produced guidance on how to handle patient complaints in order to minimise the distress caused to all parties, summarised in Box 15.9. Further guidance is offered by Leape (2007) who highlights the importance of apologising and maintaining open communication with the patient. Many people faced with a complaint are frightened of apologising in case this increases the risk of

litigation. There is no evidence to support this risk, however. Instead, studies have shown that apologising reduces the risk of litigation (or if a claim is made, the cost of the claim) (Leape, 2007). By apologising, you are showing compassion to the patient for what has happened. In addition, explaining to the patient what has happened, why it happened, and what you will do to prevent a recurrence shows respect to the patient and mitigates their suffering. In contrast, withholding information or pretending that nothing has happened shows arrogance and disrespect, destroys patients' trust in you and confirms their suspicion that something has gone wrong.

Professional negligence

One of the biggest fears a pharmacist may have during a complaint is the risk of an action for professional negligence through the civil courts or a conviction through the criminal courts under the Medicines Act (or for manslaughter). This is possible if negligence can be proved. Fortunately, civil court proceedings are rare, and criminal court proceedings even rarer. In 2002, the Chemists Defence Association received 241 claims for compensation against pharmacists or employers (Thompson, 2003). Of these, 197 involved medication-related incidents, the majority of which were dispensing errors; only 13 related to OTC sales. Although court proceedings are rare, the incidence is increasing year on year.

Charges of misconduct made by the Statutory Committee of the RPSGB are more likely than court proceedings. A charge of misconduct is even more likely if a pharmacist has made multiple mistakes, failed to address the causes of these mistakes, or appeared indifferent to the consequences of these mistakes (Appelbe & Wingfield, 2005b). Examples of pharmacists receiving reprimands (or being struck off the Pharmaceutical Register) can be found in the *Pharmaceutical Journal*. These serve as a useful warning to trainee pharmacists.

When a court determines professional negligence, three factors are taken into account (Appelbe & Wingfield, 2005b):

Box 15.9 How to manage complaints about dispensing errors

When a patient makes a complaint about a dispensing error, this must take precedence over other tasks awaiting your attention. If you are seen to take the complaint seriously, and act professionally, the complaint is less likely to escalate.

1. Establish whether the patient has taken the medicine.
2. If the patient has taken the medicine, have they been harmed by it? This may require some investigation, including contacting the local medicines information service to identify possible effects of the drug taken.
3. If the patient has been harmed, recommend an appropriate course of action (e.g. referral to the general practitioner (GP) or hospital emergency department, depending on the severity of the harm.
4. If the patient has taken the medicine, report this to their GP, irrespective of whether you believe the patient to have experienced any harm.
5. Ask to inspect the medicine that has been dispensed in error. Explain this will help you to identify what has gone wrong. Do not dispose of the medicine.
6. If an error has been made, apologise to the patient on behalf of the owner of the pharmacy and the pharmacist who made the error (even if you have made the error). This is not an admission of liability, but is likely to reduce the chance of the complaint escalating. Do not minimise the seriousness of the error, as this is likely to antagonise the patient, undermine their confidence in you, and increase the risk of litigation.
7. Explain to the patient that you need to investigate the cause of the error further, in order to prevent such an event happening again. As part of this investigation, it would be useful to speak to whoever presented the prescription in order to find out more about conditions in the pharmacy on that day (e.g. was it busy, were there any obvious distractions?) This does not need to be done immediately. Instead, it may be helpful to take contact details for the patient and contact them at a more convenient time.
8. Dispense the correct medicine against the original prescription to ensure that the patient has a safe supply.
9. If the patient wishes to make a complaint to another body, give them the contact details of the Fitness to Practise and Legal Affairs Directorate at the RPSGB and the complaints office at the local primary care trust.
10. Inform your professional indemnity insurers that you have made a mistake, in case a claim is made against you.
11. Follow the procedures in the pharmacy for reporting dispensing errors.

- Was the patient owed a duty of care?
- Did the pharmacist fail to discharge that duty?
- Has the patient suffered harm as a result?

Where all three factors are found, negligence can be proved. If a pharmacist has supplied a medicine to a patient (either on a prescription or through an OTC sale) they will be deemed to have a duty of care to that patient (this may also be true if they have refused or failed to supply a medicine that a patient has requested). A pharmacist (or pre-registration pharmacist) may be liable for prosecution for inaccurately dispensing a safe prescription, or for accurately dispensing a harmful prescription without querying it with the doctor. Examples of cases where pharmacists have been prosecuted are shown in Boxes 15.10–15.14. These cases illustrate the importance of both the professional (clinical) and accuracy (final) checks when dispensing prescriptions. In a case where a doctor has written a potentially harmful prescription that is unquestioningly dispensed by the pharmacist and causes harm to the patient, both the doctor and the pharmacist will be liable.

How is blame apportioned between prescribers and pharmacists?

In cases where a pharmacist dispenses a prescription and a patient is injured as a result, the

Box 15.10 Case study: preparing peppermint water with concentrated chloroform water

In 1998, a pharmacist and pre-registration pharmacist were charged with manslaughter after dispensing to a 3-week-old child peppermint water that had been prepared incorrectly with concentrated chloroform water (PJ, 2000). The manslaughter charges were eventually dropped but both parties were charged under the Medicines Act 1968 for supplying a medicine not of the nature or quality demanded. Two years later, the pharmacist was fined £1000 and the pre-registration pharmacist £750, based on their ability to pay. Their employer, Boots the Chemist, subsequently paid an undisclosed sum in damages to the family.

Box 15.12 Case study: dispensing an overdose of Migril

In 1982, a pharmacist dispensed Migril (ergotamine, cyclizine and caffeine) for a patient on the basis of a GP prescription (Ferguson, 1997). Neither the GP nor the pharmacist noted that the prescribed dose was an overdose and neither warned the patient about the maximum daily dose of Migril. The patient subsequently took too much Migril and developed gangrene in both legs, requiring extensive surgery.

The patient was awarded £100 000 in damages. The owner of the pharmacy was liable for 40% of these damages (£40 000) because they should have queried the maximum dose with the GP and provided adequate counselling to the patient (PJ, 1982).

Box 15.11 Case study: dispensing a dexamethasone overdose

In July 2001 a GP in the UK prescribed 28 days' supply of dexamethasone at a daily dose of 4 mg (PJ, 2006a). This was eight times the maintenance dose of 0.5 mg that the patient had taken for a number of years. The prescription was dispensed without contacting the doctor.

The increased dose was continued by the patient's regular doctor in the USA after he read the dispensing label. By the end of October, the patient developed Cushing's syndrome, requiring multiple hospital admissions and leaving her unfit for work for many months.

In this case the GP responsible for prescribing the excessive dexamethasone dose paid an undisclosed sum to the patient in an out-of-court settlement. Lloyds Pharmacy Ltd was subsequently required to pay damages because it was reasonably expected that the pharmacist should have questioned the dose increase (despite the dose being in the usual therapeutic range for dexamethasone) rather than dispensing the dexamethasone as prescribed (PJ, 2006b).

pharmacist may be considered jointly liable with the prescriber. There have been a number of cases in which pharmacists have been held jointly liable with the doctor when a patient has been injured as a result of a prescribed drug. The proportion for which the pharmacist is liable varies from case to case, depending on individual circumstances. In the cases illustrated in Boxes 15.11–15.14, the pharmacist's liability ranged from 25% to 75%, on the basis of how likely it was that the pharmacist could have averted the injury. For instance, in the case where a prescription for Amoxil was misread as Daonil (Box 15.13), the pharmacist carried 75% liability because they dispensed the wrong drug. The prescriber carried 25% liability because they wrote an illegible prescription. In the cases presented in Boxes 15.11 and 15.12, the pharmacist carries a little under half the liability because they dispensed what was prescribed, but had adequate information available to them to recognise that the prescription was an overdose. Based on this information, the pharmacist should have intervened and contacted the prescriber.

Box 15.13   Case study: dispensing Daonil instead of Amoxil

In 1983, a GP prescribed Amoxil (amoxicillin) for a patient for a chest infection. The prescription was badly written and the pharmacist mistakenly dispensed Daonil (glibenclamide, a drug used to treat non-insulin-dependent diabetes) instead of Amoxil.

The patient fell into a coma, was in hospital for 5 months and suffered irreversible brain damage as a result. Following this, he was unable to care for himself, let alone work.

The judge presiding over the case determined that the pharmacist had not been paying sufficient attention to his work. The judge felt that the dose (one to be taken three times a day instead of once a day as would be normal for Daonil) (Ferguson, 1997) and quantity prescribed should have alerted the pharmacist to the error. The pharmacist claimed he had contacted the GP to check the prescription and warned the patient's relative of the potential danger of the prescription when the Daonil was collected. There was, however, no written evidence of this.

The judge declared that the pharmacist's negligence had been triggered by the GP's poor handwriting and therefore that both parties were culpable. The patient received £138 147 in compensation, 75% from the pharmacist.

Box 15.14   Case study: dispensing an overdose of Epilim without contacting the doctor

In 1989, a GP prescribed Epilim (sodium valproate) 500 mg four times daily, which was dispensed by the pharmacist without question (Chemist & Druggist, 2000). The patient normally took Epilim 200 mg four times daily, and suffered irreversible injuries as a result of the 2.5-fold increase in dose.

The patient sued the GP, who claimed that the pharmacist should have identified the inappropriate dose increase and intervened.

The pharmacy agreed to contribute 25% towards the final damages awarded to the patient.

Summary

Supplying medicines to members of the public is a major role for pharmacists that carries a massive responsibility to ensure that their supply is safe and effective. Whilst undertaking this role, pharmacists should be aware of the numerous laws, acts and regulations that govern medicine supply in the UK. Pharmacists should ensure that they use effective risk management strategies to reduce the risk of errors occurring. This in turn reduces the risk of harm to members of the public. Even with stringent risk management strategies in place, however, errors will occur. Pharmacists need to be aware of how to deal with these errors to minimise harm to the patient, themselves and their business. In cases where patients are injured as a result of an error, pharmacists may be subject to prosecution and liable to pay damages. The amount paid will depend on the severity of injury and the assessment of shared liability between the pharmacist and prescriber.

References

Appelbe G E, Wingfield J (2005a). *Dale and Appelbe's Pharmacy Law and Ethics*, 8th edn. London: Pharmaceutical Press.

Appelbe G E, Wingfield J (2005b). Professional conduct. In: *Dale and Appelbe's Pharmacy Law and Ethics*. London: Pharmaceutical Press, 284–296.

Ashcroft D, Morecroft C, Parker D, *et al.* (2005). *Patient safety in community pharmacy: Understanding errors and managing risk*. University of Manchester. www.rpsgb.org/pdfs/patsafcommph.pdf

Butler C P (2005). Practical risk management. In: Kayne, SB, ed. *Pharmacy Business Management*. London: Pharmaceutical Press, 123–153.

Chemist & Druggist (2000). Pharmacy contributes to overdose damages. *Chemist Druggist* 253: 5.

Davis T C, Wolf M S, Bass P F III, *et al.* (2006). Literacy and misunderstanding prescription drug labels. *Ann Intern Med* 145: 887–894.

European Medicines Evaluation Agency (EMEA) (2007). *EPARs for authorised medicinal products for human use*. www.emea.europa.eu/htms/human/epar/eparintro.htm (accessed 30 May 2007).

Ferguson P R (1997). The legal liability of the community pharmacy for personal injury caused by medicinal products: (1) Liability for negligence. *Pharm J* 258: 133–135.

Leape L (2007). When things go wrong. *International Forum on Quality and Safety in Health Care.* Barcelona, Spain.

Medicines and Healthcare products Regulatory Agency (MHRA) (2006a). Marketing authorisations. Latest versions available from www.mhra.gov.uk.

Medicines and Healthcare products Regulatory Agency (MHRA) (2006b). *The supply of unlicensed relevant medicinal products for individual patients.* MHRA Guidance note no. 14. Available from www.mhra.gov.uk

PJ (1982). 40 Percent of damages in overdose case awarded against pharmacy company. *Pharm J* 228: 205.

PJ (2000). Boots pharmacist and trainee cleared of baby's manslaughter, but fined for dispensing a defective medicine. *Pharm J* 264: 390–392.

PJ (2006a). Lloyds pharmacy fighting £5m damages case. *Pharm J* 277: 440.

PJ (2006b). Lloyds pharmacy ordered to pay compensation after steroid error. *Pharm J* 277: 595.

Royal Pharmaceutical Society of Great Britain Practice Committee (2000). Guidance on counter prescribing. *Pharm J* 265: 359.

Royal Pharmaceutical Society of Great Britain (RPSGB) (2001). *Developing and implementing standard operating procedures for dispensing.* www.rpsgb.org/pdfs/sops.pdf.

RPSGB (2004). *The use of unlicensed medicines in pharmacy.* www.rpsgb.org/pdfs/factsheet5.pdf.

RPSGB (2005a). *Royal Pharmaceutical Society of Great Britain guidance on making complaints against registrants and owners of pharmacies.* www.rpsgb.org/pdfs/ftpcomplaintsprocsguide.pdf.

RPSGB (2005b). *Interim guidance from the RPSGB: Identifying and remedying pharmacist poor performance in England and Wales.* www.rpsgb.org/pdfs/pharmpoorperf0501.pdf.

RPSGB (2006a). Improving pharmacy practice. In: *Medicines, Ethics and Practice. A Guide for Pharmacists and Pharmacy Technicians*, 30th edn. London: Pharmaceutical Press, Chapter 4, 105–111.

RPSGB (2006b). *Guidance on recording interventions.* www.rpsgb.org/pdfs/recinterventionsguid.pdf.

RPSGB (2006c). *Dealing with dispensing errors.* www.rpsgb.org/pdfs/factsheet8.pdf.

RPSGB (2007). *Code of ethics for pharmacists and pharmacy technicians.* London: Royal Pharmaceutical Society of Great Britain; www.rpsgb.org/protectingthepublic/ethics/

Thompson M (2003). Trends in claims for pharmacists' errors. *Pharm J* 270: 9.

16

Major routes of drug administration

Kate E Fletcher

Aims of drug administration

The aim of drug administration is to deliver a therapeutic concentration of drug to the desired site of action. The route selected will determine time to onset of action and plasma concentration achieved (Winfield & Richards, 2004). A detailed description of drug absorption and distribution is beyond the scope of this book; however, the major routes of drugs administration will be described and discussed. *Basic Clinical Pharmacokinetics* (Winter, 2003) provides more detailed information about pharmacokinetics and pharmacodynamics.

The route chosen depends on several factors (Winfield & Richards, 2004):

- how quickly the drug's action is required
- routes available
- site of action
- properties of the drug
- desired duration of drug action.

Note: Commonly used abbreviations for each route, derived from the English or Latin for that route, are provided in brackets.

Enteral routes

Enteral routes refer to the administration of a drug via the gastrointestinal (GI) tract.

Oral

The oral route (sometimes given as p.o., from the Latin *per os*) is the most frequently used route for the administration of drugs. It involves taking a dosage form by mouth and swallowing it. The most common oral dosage forms are tablets, capsules and liquids. Drugs taken orally may have a local or systemic effect. For example, liquid antacids are taken to have a local effect by reducing pH in the stomach, whereas an antihypertensive tablet is taken to be absorbed into the circulation and thus have a systemic effect to reduce blood pressure.

Solid dosage forms taken for a systemic effect must dissolve or disperse in the stomach so that the drug can be absorbed into the blood, and exert an effect; most absorption occurs in the small intestines. Some tablets or capsules have a special coating (enteric coating) that is resistant to acid, thus preventing its breakdown in the acidic environment of the stomach, allowing it to pass into the more alkaline environment of the small intestine before dissolving and being absorbed. An enteric coat may be used to protect a drug that is made inactive by acid (e.g. omeprazole); to ensure that a tablet containing a drug that irritates the stomach lining does not dissolve in the stomach and therefore cause irritation (e.g. aspirin or prednisolone); or to protect a drug that exerts a local effect in the small or large intestine (e.g. mesalazine used for the treatment of ulcerative colitis).

The oral route has the following advantages:

- it is safe, easy and non-invasive
- tablets and capsules are easily portable
- patients can administer the drug to themselves easily

and the following disadvantages:

- relatively slow onset of action
- absorption may be affected by stomach contents
- absorption may be irregular
- drugs absorbed from the GI tract are subject to metabolism in the liver, which may reduce efficacy ('first-pass effect')
- not suitable for patients with compromised swallow (e.g. patients who have had a stroke or are unconscious or vomiting) (Winfield & Roberts, 2004).

Enteric tubes

If a patient is not able to swallow normally, it is sometimes necessary to place a tube into their GI tract, which enables food, in the form of enteral feeds (a liquid containing the complete nutritional needs of the patient, i.e. lipids, proteins, glucose, vitamins, minerals and fibre) and medications to be given. Patients might not be able to eat normally for various reasons: they may have a compromised swallow (as above), they may be unconscious (e.g. a patient in intensive care), or they may have had surgery to the oesophagus.

The most common tube used is a nasogastric (NG) tube, which is passed through the nose

and down into the stomach. Less commonly used is the nasojejunal (NJ) tube, which passes through the nose and down into the jejunum. Following the insertion of a NG tube, a small amount of the tube contents are withdrawn (aspirated) from the tube to check the pH; a pH below 5 indicates that the tube is in the stomach; a pH above 5 indicates the tube has been misplaced into the lungs. This method can be unreliable however, and the best way to check the placement of any tube is by X-ray. A radio-opaque strip renders the tube visible on X-ray. A NJ tube may be used instead of a NG tube if the patient has gastroparesis (failure of the stomach to empty into the duodenum due to lack of gastric motility), as fluids passed down a NG tube would not be absorbed.

If a tube cannot be passed through the nose, or if long-term enteral feeding is anticipated, an enterostomal tube may be placed. This entails forming a stoma (opening) through the skin of the abdomen, and placing the tube directly into the stomach or small intestine. A common example of this type of tube insertion is the

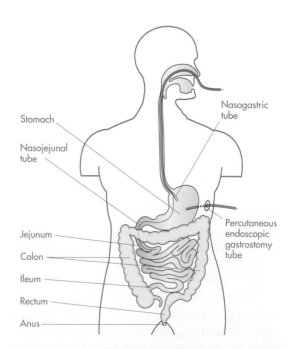

Figure 16.1 Positioning of a nasogastric tube, nasojejunal tube and a percutaneous endoscopic gastrostomy tube. A percutaneous endoscopic gastrostomy tube can also be placed in the jejunum.

percutaneous endoscopic gastrostomy (PEG): the patient is sedated or anaesthetised and, using an endoscope to visualise the interior of the stomach, the tube is passed through a stoma formed between the stomach and the skin of the abdomen. Internal and external retainers hold the tube in place. Placement of a tube into the jejunum in a similar fashion is known as a percutaneous endoscopic jejunostomy (PEJ).

Drugs may also be given via PEG and PEG tubes, but certain criteria must be considered.

- It is important not to block the tube; it is therefore important to consider whether the drug is available in a form suitable for giving via a tube (i.e. a liquid, soluble or dispersible form). Some liquid or dispersible formulations are quite thick, and so may not be suitable for tube administration, or may need to be diluted before administration. If a suitable liquid, soluble or dispersible form of a drug does not exist, it might be possible to crush a tablet form or open a capsule, mix the powder in water and, using a syringe, give the mixture via the tube. Note however that this renders the drug unlicensed, as it involves manipulation of the product.
- Some drugs (e.g. the anticonvulsant phenytoin), can interact with the enteral feed, which can reduce the efficacy of the drug. This can be avoided by stopping the feed for an interval (typically 2 hours) to allow the feed to pass from the tube site along the GI tract, giving the drug, waiting another 2 hours for the drug to leave the tube site, and then restarting the feed. This can be difficult to manage, especially if the drug is given more than once a day, because enteral feeds often run for most of the day. This can be resolved in some patients running the feed overnight, but the patient must be able to tolerate a higher flow rate for the feed.
- Drugs delivered via a PEJ directly into the small intestine can have an osmotic effect on the GI tract and cause diarrhoea. The mechanism of this is the same as that of osmotic laxatives: the drug, which has a higher osmotic potential than the GI tract contents, absorbs water and increases in volume. This increase in bulk stimulates peristalsis and therefore stimulates evacuation of the bowels.

Particular care should be taken with liquids containing sweeteners such as sorbitol, as these can have a pronounced osmotic laxative effect.

More detailed advice on administration of drugs via feeding tubes is provided in the *Handbook of Drug Administration via Enteral Feeding Tubes* (White & Bradnam, 2007) and *The NEWT Guidelines for Administration of Medication to Patients with Enteral Feeding Tubes or Swallowing Difficulties* (Smyth, 2006).

Drug delivery across mucous membranes

This includes the sublingual (SL) and buccal routes and vaginal and rectal administration.

Sublingual and buccal routes

These routes deliver drugs across the oral mucous membrane to the systemic circulation. The SL route involves placing a tablet or directing a spray under the tongue. Glyceryl trinitrate (used to treat angina) is administered in this way. For buccal delivery, the tablet is placed between the upper lip and gum. This route is used to administer prochlorperazine (used to treat nausea and vomiting). A solid dosage form placed sublingually or buccally will dissolve in the saliva and the drug is then able to cross the mucous membrane of the mouth into the circulation. A spray directed under the tongue will disperse into the saliva and then the drug will be absorbed in the same way.

The buccal route may be used to give a more prolonged action than with the SL route. Drugs such as nicotine, in the form of nicotine replacement therapy, can be formulated as a lozenge or chewing gum that is sucked or chewed periodically, and rested in the buccal cavity when not in use.

The advantages of the SL and buccal routes are:

- fast absorption and onset of action
- avoiding of first-pass effect (see above)

- can be used in unconscious patients
- as dosage form is not swallowed, antiemetics such as prochlorperazine can be given buccally.

The disadvantages of the SL and buccal routes are:

- poor adherence if the medication has unpleasant taste
- some drugs are ineffective if swallowed because of metabolism by the liver (e.g. glyceryl trinitrate)
- route is not effective if patient has a dry mouth, as saliva is required to dissolve dosage form to facilitate absorption (Winfield & Roberts, 2004)

Rectal administration (Latin *per rectum*; PR)

Two main dosage forms can be used to deliver drugs to the rectum: suppositories and enemas (liquid or foam). In the UK, most drugs delivered rectally are for local action, for example steroids in inflammatory bowel disease; laxatives for constipation. Rectal administration can also be useful for systemic drug delivery in situations where other routes are not safe or possible, such as giving diazepam during an epileptic seizure.

The rectal route is generally not popular in the UK as many patients do not feel comfortable with the idea of administering medication this way. It is used more frequently in other parts of Europe such as France and Germany.

The blood supply to the rectum is composed of three veins, two of which drain directly into the systemic circulation, and one directly to the liver. Therefore, not all the drug absorbed in the rectum will undergo first-pass metabolism, which may increase bioavailability compared with other routes (Winfield & Roberts, 2004).

There are currently two schools of thought about the best way to insert a suppository: rounded end first, as indeed they are designed to be inserted, for ease and comfort; or blunt end first, which some practitioners believe aids retention in the rectum. It may well be easier for patients to self-administer round-end first; in hospital, however, most suppositories are inserted by nurses, and it is equally easy for

nurses to insert them round- or blunt-end first (Wright *et al.,* 2006). Whichever method is used, it is important that the suppository is retained in the rectum for long enough for it to melt, so the drug can be absorbed. As enemas are liquid or foam, the drug is already in a form which makes it available for absorption.

Absorption from the rectum can be erratic and unreliable, so this route is not suitable for drugs with a narrow therapeutic index (see Box 16.1). The rectal route may also be contraindicated in patients after recent colorectal surgery because of the risk of rupturing anastomoses (see Box 16.1).

The rectal route has the following advantages:

- useful for local administration of drug to the rectum
- may be used when other routes unavailable (e.g. during an epileptic seizure)

and disadadvantages

- patients may not be keen to use this route
- absorption is erratic
- less convenient than oral route
- suppository or enema must be retained in rectum long enough for drug to be absorbed
- some rectal dosage forms might be irritant and can only be used for a limited time (e.g. carbamazepine suppositories).

Vaginal (Latin per vagina; PV)

The formulations most commonly used to deliver a drug vaginally are the pessary, vaginal tablet, cream or ointment. This route is usually used for local action of the drug (e.g. anti-fungal pessary to treat vaginal candidiasis; see Box 16.1).

Pessaries and vaginal tablets are often supplied with an applicator to aid insertion; applicators should be used in pregnancy because of the risk of miscarriage or induction of premature labour due to mechanical stimulation of the cervix.

Topical drug delivery

Topical drug delivery refers to administration of drugs to the skin or mucous membranes (Hall &

Morton 2002). There are several topical routes: ears, eyes, nose, skin and transdermal.

Delivery of drugs to the ear

The main indications for the use of drops in the ears are for treatment of otitis externa or otitis media (see Box 16.1), and to soften ear wax. The drugs are used for a local effect. Examples are anti-inflammatory agents such as corticosteroids (e.g. prednisolone, betamethasone) to treat otitis externa; antimicrobials such as gentamicin to treat otitis media; sodium bicarbonate and oils such as almond or olive oil are used to soften ear wax.

Technique for application of ear drops

The usual dose of drops used in the ear is two or three drops, the frequency depending on the drug being administered. The person administering the drops should first wash their hands. The patient's head should be tipped sideways with the ear to be treated uppermost; ideally they should lie down. Instil two or three drops into the ear, taking care not to touch the tip of the bottle on the skin, as this will increase the risk of contaminating the ear drops. The patient's head should remain in position for a few minutes to allow the drops to disperse into the ear and be absorbed.

Delivery of drugs to the eye

Two formulations are used to deliver drugs to the eye: drops and ointment. Drops are usually easier to apply; ointment is suitable for use at night as it may have a prolonged contact time, but it can be more difficult to apply and may interfere with vision for longer than eye drops, because of the usually greasy nature of the formulation. Absorption of the drug occurs through the epithelium of the conjunctival sac (Rang *et al.*, 2007).

Eye preparations can be used to treat dry eyes, infection, inflammation and glaucoma (see Box 16.1), or to facilitate eye examination or procedures, for instance, mydriatics to dilate the pupil; local anaesthetics prior to minor surgery.

Technique for application of eye drops

The dose is usually one drop – any more will flood out of the eye and be wasted. Frequency depends on the drug being administered. The person administering the drops should first wash their hands. If the patient is wearing contact lenses, they should remove them. The patient's head should be tipped back – ideally they should sit or lie down – and they should look upwards. Gently pull down the lower lid of the eye to be treated, to form a pouch. The patient should look away from the dropper, without moving their head, to stop them blinking too soon. Squeeze one drop into the pouch and gently release eyelid. Be careful not to touch the tip of the bottle on the eye, as this will increase the risk of contaminating the eye drops. The patient should keep the eye closed for about 30 seconds to allow the drop to disperse over the eye and be absorbed. Wipe away any excess with a clean tissue.

If more medication is to be administered into the eye at the same time of day, allow about 5 minutes between applications of the products to allow time for absorption. If the drugs are administered too closely together, the drops will overflow the eye and the efficacy of each drop will be reduced. A device called an autodropper is available for patients who have difficulty administering eye drops to themselves, or they may find that resting the bottle across the nose makes application easier.

Technique for the application of eye ointment

The process for application of eye ointment is broadly similar to that described above for the administration of eye drops. A line of ointment should be squeezed along the inside of the pouch formed with the lower eyelid, being careful not to touch the tip of the tube on the eye (as this will increase the risk of contaminating the ointment). The patient should close their eye, and allow the ointment to disperse over the eye. Blinking several times will help spread the ointment.

If drops and ointment are to be applied at the same time of day, administer the eye drop about 5 minutes before the ointment. This allows the eye drop to be absorbed before the ointment is applied, reducing the risk of the drop being displaced by the ointment.

Patients may experience stinging when eye drops or ointment are applied, but this is usually transient. However, they should be advised to see their doctor if the stinging continues or redness and itching develop, as this could indicate that they are allergic to the preparation. The allergen could be the drug or one of the excipients. The preservative is often the cause of an allergy to eye preparations. The risk of developing an allergy is increased by very frequent administration (e.g. every hour in severe infections) because of repeated exposure to the preservative in the drops. Some eye drops are also available as preservative-free formulations; many prescribers will choose these formulations for patients who use the drops frequently, to reduce the risk of developing an allergy. However, preservative-free drops are not used as a first choice for several reasons: they tend to be more expensive than drops with preservatives; they may not be commercially available and therefore an unlicensed product must be used; they often have to be stored in the fridge or may need to be frozen, making transport and storage difficult and expensive; they often have a short shelf life (especially unlicensed products) and so may have to be disposed of 24 hours after opening; they may be packaged in single dose units, which makes them bulky, and these must be used once only and then discarded.

Delivery of drugs to the nose

Drugs may be delivered to the nose using drops or a spray. Currently there are few indications for topical delivery to the nose; some patients benefit from drops or sprays to treat rhinitis or to reduce nasal polyps (see Box 16.1). More recently, however, drugs for systemic action are being developed as intranasal formulations, exploiting the good blood supply to the nasal tissue. One example is desmopressin (an analogue of vasopressin (antidiuretic hormone) used in the treatment of conditions such diabetes insipidus). It is thought that absorption of the drug occurs across the mucosa covering nasal-related lymphoid tissue (Rang *et al.*, 2007).

Technique for the application of nasal drops

The patient should blow their nose gently, to make sure it is clear. The person administering the drops should wash their hands. The patient's head should be tipped back. Hold the dropper just above the nose and squeeze in three of four drops, being careful not to touch the dropper on the nose, as this will increase the risk of contaminating the drops. The patient should keep the head tipped back for a few minutes to help the drops run to the back of the nose.

Skin

Creams, ointments, lotions, gels and powders can be used to deliver drugs to the skin for local action. Drugs delivered in this way include corticosteroids used to treat eczema and antimicrobials used to treat a skin infection. Emollient preparations, used to soothe and soften the skin, such as aqueous cream or Diprobase, do not deliver any drug to the skin but contain ingredients that help hydrate and soften the skin, such as white soft paraffin and liquid paraffin. These are used for dry skin conditions such as eczema and psoriasis.

The advantage of drug delivery to the skin is that local effects are achieved. The disadvantages are:

- some areas are hard to reach (e.g. the back)
- some preparations are messy (e.g. ointments or lotions) or stain clothing and bedding (e.g. dithranol, coal tar)
- some preparations may cause irritation when applied, especially in conditions such as eczema.

Transdermal drug delivery

Systemic drug action can be obtained by delivering the drug using a transdermal system, such as a patch or gel. Transdermal means 'across the skin'. Patches are used to deliver drugs such as hormones (e.g. oestradiol), analgesics (e.g. fentanyl) and glyceryl trinitrate to the systemic circulation. As the drug enters directly into the blood stream, the first-pass effect is avoided.

Patches are designed to deliver a drug over a sustained period, ranging from a few hours to 7 days. Drug activity is sustained for several hours after the patch is removed because of a reservoir of drug that forms in the skin.

Advantages of transdermal drug delivery are:

- prolonged drug delivery that is convenient for patient – the patch can be changed every few days, rather than taking an oral preparation several times a day
- constant rate of drug delivery
- non-invasive.

Disadvantages are:

- slow onset of action – some drugs may take up to 12 hours to reach therapeutic levels
- fixed dose of drug, therefore additional routes may be required (e.g. additional doses of analgesia for breakthrough pain) (see Box 16.1)
- limited number of drugs can be given via this route.

Inhalation drugs

The lungs have a very large surface area and rich blood supply, making them an ideal site for the absorption of drugs; however, because of the difficulty of delivering drugs to the lungs, most drugs delivered by inhalation are for local action – for the treatment of respiratory diseases such as asthma and chronic obstructive pulmonary disease. Drugs delivered in this way include corticosteroids (e.g. beclometasone and fluticasone) and beta-agonists (e.g. salbutamol and terbutaline). Local delivery of these drugs reduces the occurrence of side-effects; because the drug is delivered directly to the site of action, a much smaller dose can be used to exert the same effect a larger dose would produce if given systemically, therefore reducing systemic side-effects.

Drugs inhaled for a systemic action have for many years been restricted to volatile and gaseous anaesthetics; however, a recent development has been the delivery of insulin by inhaler. Insulin is a polypeptide and therefore cannot be taken orally, as it would be inactivated by stomach acid and digestive enzymes. Consequently, administration has been restricted to subcutaneous injection or intravenous infusion. A new inhaled formulation therefore offers a less invasive route which may be particularly useful for patients who are needle phobic or have difficulty injecting themselves.

Drugs delivered to the lung for local action are usually administered as an aerosol, using either a small handheld inhaler device, or a nebuliser. Several types of handheld inhaler are available, with different mechanisms: the pressurised metered-dose inhaler (MDI), the breath-actuated metered-dose powder inhaler (Turbohaler), breath-actuated pressurised MDI, e.g. Easi-Breathe. Instructions on how to use these devices are provided in the patient information leaflet packaged with each device. A nebuliser makes an aerosol by blowing air or oxygen through a solution of a drug, and delivering the aerosol to the patient's mouth for inhalation via a mask or mouthpiece (Marcovitch, 2005). Nebulisers are used in two situations: by patients with very severe symptoms, as the dose of drug delivered is higher than that delivered by an inhaler; or when a patient is acutely unwell during an asthma attack or infection that exacerbates their symptoms, and needs a higher dose but also is too unwell to use an inhaler properly.

A spacer device can make an MDI easier to use. A spacer is a plastic chamber with a hole at one end into which the inhaler nozzle fits; at the other end is a mouth piece with a one-way valve. The inhaler is actuated into the chamber, and the patient breathes through the mouthpiece to inhale the drug aerosol. Spacers may increase drug delivery to the lungs by 50% (Wright *et al.*, 2006).

The advantages of the inhaled route are:

- large surface area and rich blood supply for absorption
- direct delivery to lung tissue for local action
- smaller dose used therefore fewer systemic side-effects.

The disadvantages of the inhaled route are that inhaler devices can be difficult to use properly, therefore reducing efficacy, and equipment such as spacer devices and nebulisers are not very portable.

Parenteral routes

Parenteral refers to administration by injection. The most commonly used parenteral routes will be discussed in this section.

Intravenous (IV)

The IV route involves injection of a drug directly into the venous circulation. The bioavailability (see Box 16.1) of a drug given IV is 100%. It is the fastest way to administer a drug: a bolus injection (a small-volume injection given over less than 5 minutes) will produce very high drug concentrations, first of all in the right side of the heart and lungs, and then the systemic circulation (Rang *et al.*, 2007).

Large volumes (> 20 mL) to be given IV are given by infusion, which may take from 10 minutes to 24 hours (i.e. continuous). Continuous infusions are used to deliver large volumes of fluids to rehydrate and maintain hydration in patients who are acutely dehydrated or unable to take fluids by other routes. Infusions are also used to deliver drugs that need to be diluted to avoid irritating the veins, drugs that need to be given slowly to avoid side-effects, and drugs that have a short elimination half-life (see Box 16.1) and so need to be delivered frequently or continuously to maintain action.

Access into the venous system must be achieved in order to administer drugs IV. For single injections, a needle is inserted into a superficial vein in the internal flexure of the elbow. If drugs are to be given IV for several days, a cannula will be placed into a superficial vein either in the internal flexure of the elbow or on the back of the hand. A central venous catheter can be used if long-term IV access is required.

The advantages of IV administration are:

- rapid delivery and onset of action
- 100% bioavailability
- large volumes may be given.

The disadvantages are:

- it is painful and invasive
- risk of infection at injection site

- patient is more dependent on nurses
- patient mobility reduced when infusions are running
- injectable formulations of some drugs are more expensive than oral formulations
- risk of acute overdose if drug given too quickly.

Subcutaneous (SC)

The SC route may be used to administer a drug by injection, or to administer large volumes of fluids by infusion.

An SC injection is given into the tissue directly under the skin, most commonly on the abdomen or the upper arms. Because the fluid has to be forced into the tissue, the maximum volume that can be administered by this route is usually 1 mL – it can be painful and difficult to administer more than this to one site. Volumes of more than 1 mL must be given in multiple smaller volumes at different sites.

Drugs given SC are absorbed more quickly compared with the oral route. The rate of absorption is related to the blood flow at the injection site; therefore, a site that is warm, has a good blood supply, or is massaged after injection, will have a higher blood flow and the rate of drug absorption will be increased. Conversely, drug absorption will be slower from an injection site that is cold or has a poor blood supply.

SC infusions are used to administer 2–3 litres of fluids a day to patients who are dehydrated and unable to take adequate fluids orally, but who do not require rapid fluid replacement. (The IV route would be used in this situation as faster infusion rates can be used.) This is also known as hypodermoclysis. Examples in which hypodermoclysis may be used include patients who have had a stroke and may not be able to swallow safely, and terminally ill patients who require fluids as part of palliative care (see Box 16.1). Commonly used sites are the abdomen and thigh. Fluids given by SC infusion should be isotonic to extracellular fluid. Examples include 0.9% or 0.45% sodium chloride solution and 5% glucose, although this should be limited to 2 litres in 24 hours and maximum rate of 2 mL/minute, as higher rates and concentrations may lead to shock. The following fluids are not suitable for SC infusion:

- colloids
- solutions containing potassium concentrations above 40 mmol/litre
- solutions with a pH below 5.3 or above 8.2
- glucose solutions stronger than 5%
- solutions with osmolality above 280 mOsmol/kg (Wright *et al.*, 2006).

Infusion sites should be monitored regularly (several times a day, and at least at every bag change) and changed if any of the following occur: pain, irritation, site becomes inflamed, white or hard, or blood is seen in giving set, as these might indicate an infection (Wright *et al.*, 2006).

The enzyme hyaluronidase is sometimes used to enhance permeation of fluids into the subcutaneous tissues. It breaks down the intercellular matrix, and therefore increases diffusion and drug absorption (*British National Formulary*; Rang *et al.*, 2007)

The advantages of the SC route are that access is easier than IV, and absorption is relatively uniform. The disadvantages are discomfort and pain, risk of infection at the injection site and injections are limited to small volumes.

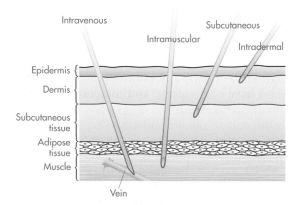

Intravenous

Intramuscular

Subcutaneous

Intradermal

Epidermis
Dermis
Subcutaneous tissue
Adipose tissue
Muscle
Vein

Figure 16.2 Drugs can be injected into the skin, subcutaneous fat, muscle or a vein.

Intramuscular (IM)

This is an injection into a muscle. Common sites are the upper arm (deltoid muscle), thigh (vastus lateralis) and buttocks (gluteal muscles). The maximum injection volume depends on the site used: 5 mL for the thigh; 2 mL for the deltoid. Larger volumes must be given in several smaller volumes at different sites, otherwise they will not be effectively absorbed, and can lead to abscess formation (Wright *et al.*, 2006). IM injections are avoided in children as the muscles are not adequately developed, and should not be given to patients with deranged blood clotting, as a haematoma is likely to develop (see Box 16.1).

As with SC injections, absorption of drug following IM injection is increased by increasing the blood flow; therefore exercising the muscle after an injection will increase absorption, but this may or may not be desirable, depending on the drug.

The major advantage of the IM route is that access is easier than with IV administration. The disadvantages are that it is painful, there is a risk of infection at the injection site and injections are limited to small volumes.

Intradermal

This route is used for diagnostic testing of allergy and immunity, and also to administer some vaccines. It involves injection of a small volume, typically 0.1 mL, between the epidermis and the dermis. Absorption is slow as the drug must diffuse through this tissue to enter the circulation (Wright *et al.*, 2006).

Intrathecal (IT)

This involves injection into the subarachnoid space via a lumbar puncture (see Box 16.1). This route is potentially dangerous, as a needle must be placed near the spinal cord, and incorrect placement can lead to permanent damage and paralysis. It is used to treat some central nervous system (CNS) infections, such as meningitis, and may be used to administer local anaesthesia,

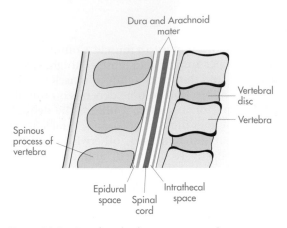

Figure 16.3 Intrathecal administration involves injection into the subarachnoid space of the spine via a lumbar puncture. Drugs, particularly local anaesthetics, can also be injected into the epidural space.

or to administer chemotherapeutic drugs to prevent relapse of certain childhood leukaemias in the CNS (Rang *et al.*, 2007).

A great deal of care must be taken when administering a drug by IT injections. As well as the risk of incorrect placement of the needle, adminstration of the wrong drug via this route can prove fatal, as has unfortunately happened on several occasions when chemotherapeutic drugs have been mixed up. In one case the vinca alkaloid vincristine was given IT, resulting in the slow death of the recipient. Vincristine is safe when given IV, but causes irreversible damage to brain tissue. As a result of these errors, strict policies and procedures are now in place in UK hospitals to prevent this happening again (Department of Health, 2003).

Epidural

This involves injecting a drug into the epidural space around the spinal column via a lumbar puncture (see Figure 16.3). It carries similar risks to an IT injection because of the close proximity of the needle to the spinal cord. The most common use of the epidural route is to administer a local anaesthetic to women during labour.

Intraperitoneal (IP)

This involves injection or infusion of drugs or fluid directly into the peritoneal cavity, via a catheter placed through the abdominal wall. The peritoneal cavity contains the abdominal organs, and is lined by a membrane called the peritoneum. This route is used in patients undergoing continuous ambulatory peritoneal dialysis (CAPD), to administer dialysis fluids, and antibiotics in the treatment of infections (i.e. peritonitis that can occur as a result of the CAPD).

Intra-articular (IA)

This refers to injection into the synovial fluid of a joint cavity, used for the administration of anti-inflammatory drugs such as the corticosteroids triamcinolone and methylprednisolone in the local treatment of rheumatoid arthritis. Injection volume differs according to the size of the joint (Wright *et al.*, 2006). IA injections can be painful, and there is a risk of damaging the cartilage. They should not be given if there is infection in the joint or surrounding tissue (Wright *et al.*, 2006).

Intra-osseous (IO)

This route is used in children under 6 years of age and requires a special needle to be placed into the tibia (thigh bone), with the tip extending into the marrow cavity. This cavity is continuous with the venous circulation, so provides a route for administering fluids and drugs when the IV route is difficult to obtain and when rapid infusions are necessary, such as in trauma. Infusions must be administered under gentle pressure, which can be exerted by hand using a syringe, or by inflating a blood pressure cuff around an infusion bag (Vreede *et al.*, 2000; Wright *et al.*, 2006).

Box 16.1   Definitions of terms relating to drug administration

anastomoses: the surgical connection of separate or severed tubular hollow organs to form a continuous channel, as between two parts of the intestine

bioavailability: the proportion of drug administered that is available at the site of action

breakthrough pain: intermittent pain experienced despite the patient receiving regular analgesia; may occur for example on movement or during dressing changes. Extra doses of analgesia may be given to alleviate this pain

colloids: solutions containing molecules with large molecular weights that contribute to the oncotic pressure at the microvascular endothelium; used mainly for plasma expansion; examples include gelatine solutions (Gelofusine, Haemaccel); starches (hexastarch, pentastarch); dextrans (dextran 40 or 70); albumin 5% or 20%

continuous ambulatory peritoneal dialysis (CAPD): a renal replacement therapy (dialysis) method for removing waste such as urea and potassium from the blood, as well as excess fluid, when the kidneys are incapable of this (i.e. in renal failure)

glaucoma: loss of visual field associated with cupping of the optic disc and optic nerve damage; it is often associated with increased intra-ocular pressure

half-life: the time taken to remove 50% of a drug from the plasma

haematoma: a solid swelling of clotted blood within the tissues

lumbar puncture: the insertion of a hollow needle beneath the arachnoid membrane of the spinal cord in the lumbar region to withdraw cerebrospinal fluid for diagnostic purposes or to administer medication

therapeutic index: the ratio between the toxic dose and the therapeutic dose of a drug, used as a measure of the relative safety of the drug for a particular treatment. A narrow therapeutic index indicates a small difference between therapeutic and toxic doses

nasal polyps: growths of a soft jelly-like character: they arise from chronic inflammation associated with allergic rhinitis, chronic sinusitis, asthma and aspirin misuse. (Marcovitch, 2005)

otitis externa: inflammation of the meatal skin of the ear (the skin of the ear canal)

otitis media: infection of the middle ear

palliative care: treatment given to improve the quality of life of patients and families who face life-threatening illness, by providing pain and symptom relief and spiritual and psychosocial support from diagnosis to the end of life and bereavement

rhinitis: inflammation of the mucous membrane of the nose

subarachnoid space: the space between the arachnoid and the pia mater, two of the three membranes covering the brain and spinal cord (the third is the dura mater); this space is filled with cerebrospinal fluid

vaginal candidiasis: a fungal infection of the vagina, characterised by vulval itchiness and a whitish, creamy discharge from the vagina, caused by *Candida* species, particularly *Candida albicans*; also known as 'thrush'

References

Hall J M, Morton I K M (2002). *The Royal Society of Medicine: Medicines*. London: The Medicines Guide Ltd.

Department of Health (2003). *HSC 2003/010 – Updated national guidance on the safe administration of intrathecal chemotherapy*. Available via www.dh.gov.uk/en/Publicationsandstatistics/Lettersandcirculars/Healthservicecirculars/DH_4064931.

Marcovitch H, ed (2005). *Black's Medical Dictionary*, 41st edn. London: A&C Black Publishers.

Rang H, Dale M, Ritter J, Flower R (2007). *Rang and Dale's Pharmacology*, 6th edn. Oxford: Churchill Livingstone.

Smyth J (2006). *The NEWT Guidelines for Administration of Medication to Patients with Enteral Feeding Tubes or Swallowing Difficulties*. North East Wales NHS Trust.

Vreede E, Bulatovic A, Rosseel P, Lassalle X (2000). Intraosseous infusion. *Update in Anaesthesia* 12: 38–40.

White R, Bradnam V (2007). *Handbook of Drug Administration via Enteral Feeding Tubes*. London: Pharmaceutical Press.

Winfield A J, Richards R M E, eds (2004). *Pharmaceutical Practice*, 3rd edn. Oxford: Churchill Livingstone.

Winter M E, ed. (2003). *Basic Clinical Pharmacokinetics*, 4th edn. Lippincott Williams and Wilkins.

Wright J, Gray A H, Goodey V (2006). *Clinical Pharmacy*. London: Pharmaceutical Press.

Glossary of terms commonly used in Pharmacy Practice

Accreditation training
Training to acquire the list of skills that a dispensing technician should be competent to carry out in order to become an accredited technician. As part of the training, student technicians produce a portfolio of evidence to demonstrate their competence.

Accuracy check
The final check that a pharmacist (or appropriately qualified technician if a prescription has already been clinically checked by a pharmacist) makes to ensure the dispensed medicinal product is the same as that requested by the prescriber on a prescription.

Active listening
This involves giving the person who is speaking to you your full attention and includes the use of both verbal encouragers (such as 'yes', 'aha' and 'mm') and non-verbal acknowledgements such as nodding, smiling and receptive body language.

Acute trust
See NHS acute trust.

Adherence
The extent to which a person's behaviour – taking medication, following a diet, and/or executing lifestyle changes – corresponds with agreed recommendations from a health professional.

Administering
The process of giving a medicine to a patient.

Advanced service
The middle tier of service provision under the new Pharmacy Contract, which includes services that can be commissioned from community pharmacies by primary care trusts according to the needs of the local population.

Adverse drug reaction (ADR)
An unintended unpleasant reaction to a drug which occurs at doses used in humans for prophylaxis, diagnosis or therapy of disease, or for the modification of physiological function.

ADRs can range in severity from a minor inconvenience (such as a headache) to death.

Adverse-effect profile
The range of ADRs that are known to occur with a medicinal product.

Adverse event
An event that results in patient harm; this could include an ADR or may be caused by an error on the part of a health professional or the patient.

Agenda for change
Process through which the employment contracts for non-medical NHS employees were reviewed, with a view to streamlining pay scales and conditions of employment.

Ambulance Trusts
Thirteen trusts that provide transport and emergency care for patients, including the 999 ambulance service and transport for patients to hospital appointments if required.

Anaesthetise
Render a patient unable to feel pain; this may be local anaesthesia, in which a local anesthetic is applied (either to the skin or by injection)

	to a specific area of the body, or general anaesthesia, in which a patient is put into a deep sleep using a general anaesthetic.
Analgesic	Medication used to relieve pain (painkiller).
Anastomosis	The surgical connection of separate or severed tubular hollow organs to form a continuous channel, such as two parts of the intestine.
Anticoagulant clinic	A place where patients taking blood-thinning medications (such as warfarin) have their blood tested. The blood sample is used to check the international normalised ratio (INR), which is a measure of clotting ability.
Antiemetic	Medication used to stop vomiting.
Apothecary	Apothecary (from the Latin *apothecarius:* a keeper of an otheca (a store)) is an historical name for a medical practitioner who formulates and dispenses *materia medica* to physicians, surgeons and patients – a role now served by a pharmacist.
Arterial aneurysm	A weakening in the wall of an artery, causing it to stretch under the pressure of the blood flow.
Aspirate	To withdraw fluid by the use of suction, usually by using a syringe (e.g. the liquid contents in the stomach can be aspirated by drawing them up through a tube inserted down through the nose into the stomach, using a large syringe). Also refers to the inhalation of fluid or stomach contents into the lungs, and to the withdrawal of cells or fluid from the body, for instance from a cyst.
Assistant technical officer (ATO)	An unqualified member of the pharmacy support staff (usually working in a hospital pharmacy) who is able to perform a limited number of tasks under the supervision of a more senior member of the pharmacy staff.
Audit	A process of comparing what currently happens in practice with what should be happening, with a view to improving the delivery of services.
Bioavailability	The relationship between the dose administered and the concentration of unchanged drug in plasma, usually expressed as a percentage.
Biotechnology	Laboratory-based techniques being developed in biological research, such as processes using recombinant DNA technology or tissue culture.
'Black listed' medicines	Medicines that cannot be prescribed on an NHS prescription.
'Black triangle' drugs	Medicinal products that have recieved marketing authorisation in the past 2 years (indicated in the *British National Formulary* and on their packaging by a black triangle). Any suspected adverse effects that occur in patients taking these drugs should be reported to the MHRA (see below) via the Yellow Card Scheme.
Blame-orientated approach	An approach which, when an error occurs, focuses on the individual responsible for the error and often involves punishing that individual, for example through suspension or dismissal.
Bolus injection	A small volume of fluid injected over a short period of time (up to 5 minutes).
Borderline substances	A list of products that have been defined by the Advisory Committee for Borderline Substances as medicinal products and that can be prescribed on an NHS prescription.
Brand-to-generic switches	The process of changing a prescription from a branded medication to the equivalent generic medication, which may result in cost savings to the NHS.
Branded medication	A medicine where the formula and mode of manufacture are the property of the manufacturer.

British National Formulary	A compendium of the licensed medicinal products and appliances that are available for prescription in the UK, published every 6 months (includes clinical indications, recommended doses, preparations, prices, licensed category, adverse drug reactions, cautions and contra-indications); often referred to as the *BNF*; medicines for children are described in the *C-BNF*.
British Pharmaceutical conference	Annual meeting for pharmacists and other scientists working within the pharmaceutical industry, where research is presented and professional issues discussed.
Buccal	Administration of a medication by placing it in the mouth between the gum and top lip or cheek.
Bulk medication	Large quantity of medication provided in large bottles, which are then dispensed into smaller quantities to individual patients; also known as bulk stock.
Bulk stock	*See* Bulk medication.
Care trusts	Organisations that provide a link between local government authorities and primary care trusts to improve the delivery of social care to patients.
Caution	Conditions where care should be exercised in using a particular drug (e.g. existing disease state).
Central venous catheter	An intravenous line that is inserted into a large vein above the heart, through which injections and infusions of drugs and blood products may be given, and blood samples withdrawn, without causing pain to the patient.
Ceramic slab	A slab made of a ceramic material upon which creams and ointments are made (commonly known as a tile).
Chemist's nostrum	*See* Nostrum.
Chief Medical Officer (CMO)	Principal medical adviser to the Government on health care in England.
Chief Pharmaceutical Officer (CPO)	Professional lead for Pharmacy at the Department of Health.
Child-resistant closure (CRC)	Lids or other seals on primary packaging of medication that are designed to be difficult for children to open, such as lids which have to be pushed down before they can be turned.
Clic Loc®	A brand of CRC commonly used on bottles.
Clinical check	The process of evaluating a prescription for the clinical appropriateness for use in an individual patient. This is ideally done when a prescription is first received by a pharmacist.
Clinical governance	A series of tools that help pharmacists (and other health professionals) to deliver a high-quality service to patients, with a focus on continually improving the quality of service delivered.
Clinical management plan (CMP)	A plan for the treatment of an individual patient that specifies which medications a supplementary prescriber can prescribe and under which circumstances; the CMP is agreed with both the patient and their doctor.
Clinical pharmacy	The activities and services undertaken by a clinical pharmacist to ensure rational and appropriate use of medicines; may take place in many settings, such as hospitals, community pharmacies, nursing homes and clinics.
Clinical training rotation	Term used to describe the training of junior pharmacists in a number of different clinical specialities by working in different clinical areas on a rotational basis.

Closed question	A question that can only be answered with a small number of responses, such as yes or no.
Closure	The lid or other method of sealing a medicinal product in the primary packaging.
Colloid	A suspension containing molecules with large molecular weights.
Colorectal surgery	Surgery on the lower part of the intestine – the colon and rectum.
Commissioner	The person who is responsible for commissioning health services within a primary care trust.
Commissioning	The process by which primary care trusts and general practices purchase health services for the general population that they serve.
Community pharmacist	A pharmacist working in the community sector of pharmacy.
Community pharmacy	A premises registered with the RPSGB (*see* below) for the provision of pharmaceutical services to the general public; a term used to describe the skills specifically used by a community pharmacist in their day-to-day work.
Complementary medicines	A general term for an extensive list of medical systems that differ from allopathic (Western) medicine, including acupuncture, Ayurvedic, tribal traditional medicine, herbal or phytotherapeutic, homoeopathic and other treatments. Complementary medicine is not the same as holistic medicine.
Compliance	The extent to which a person's behaviour – taking medications, following a recommended diet or executing lifestyle changes – coincides with medical or health advice.
Composition	The proportion and combination of elements or components that form a substance.
Compounding	The process of combining more than one chemical agent to produce a medicinal product.
Compromised swallow	Patients who have difficulty swallowing are described as having a 'compromised swallow' (e.g. after a stroke), and may require non-oral dosage forms.
Concordance	Describes an equal relationship between a patient and a health professional in which decisions about health care, including medication taking, are made in partnership, with each person contributing their own type of expertise and both parties agreeing on the final decision.
Confections	A sweetened medicinal product; a sweet preparation.
Conical measure	A type of laboratory glassware that consists of a conical cup with a notch on the top to allow for the easy pouring of liquids; conical measures have graduated markings on the side to allow easy and accurate measurement of volumes.
Conserve	A product that has been preserved with sugar.
Continuing professional development (CPD)	The process of life-long learning that will soon be mandatory for pharmacists who wish to continue to practise in the UK.
Contraindication	A medical condition or factor that increases the risk involved in using a drug to the extent that the risks are likely to outweigh the benefits; The risk–benefit ratio of using the drug must be considered in individual patients and may prohibit the use of the drug.
Controlled drug (CD)	A medicinal product that is categorised in Schedules 1–5 of the Misuse of Drugs Regulations 2001 because it is considered to be dangerous or otherwise harmful.

Controlled drug (CD) register	A record of CDs that are kept in a pharmacy or hospital ward, where they have been received from, and who they have been supplied to. The number of dose units in the register must agree with the number of physical dose units in the pharmacy.
Cost-effectiveness	The relative cost of a treatment compared with the therapeutic effect it will have. Ideally, a treatment should be low cost and provide a strong benefit to the majority of patients it is intended for.
Counter prescribing	The process of recommending over-the-counter (OTC) treatments (or other non-prescription remedies) for patients.
Critical care	The area of the hospital where patients who require intensive care are treated (such as the intensive care/therapy init (ICU/ITU)).
Critical event	An occasion where something significant has occurred that is outside normal experience. The occurrence can be positive (such as unusually excellent patient service) or negative (such as an adverse event resulting in patient harm).
Decongestant	A medication used to relieve a blocked nose.
Demijohn	A large narrow-necked bottle made of glass or earthenware, usually encased in wickerwork.
Dental Practitioners' Formulary	A list of medicinal products that can be prescribed by a dentist on an NHS prescription.
Department of Health (DH)	Government department that runs the NHS in England.
Dependent prescriber	*See* Supplementary prescriber.
Deranged blood clotting	An abnormality in the ability of the blood to clot. This is indicated by abnormal blood test results, and the presence of signs such as bruising and bleeding gums (blood clotting is decreased) or an increased tendency to clot, producing clots in the legs (deep venous thrombosis).
Deregulated	A term used to describe the down-grading in classification of a medication from prescription only (POM) to a pharmacy medicine ('P'), or from 'P' to general sales list (GSL).
Destruction of old pharmaceuticals (DOOP) bins	Bins used in pharmacies to contain drugs that need to be destroyed (e.g. out-of-date medications, and medications returned by patient).
Diagnosis	The identification of a condition or disease state that a patient has.
Diploma in clinical pharmacy	A postgraduate qualification available to both hospital and community pharmacists that provides in-depth knowledge on how to manage the use of drugs in patients with a variety of disease states.
Disintegration testing	Measurement of the time taken for a dosage form (e.g. tablet) to fully break apart under specific experimental conditions. Disintegration is often required for the drug to be released and absorbed.
Dispensary	The area within a pharmacy where medicines are dispensed.
Dispensary receptionist	Member of the pharmacy support staff who answers the telephone and greets patients and health professionals who visit the hospital pharmacy.
Dispensing	The process of supplying a medicine to a patient in accordance with the directions on a prescription.
Dispensing assistant	Member of the pharmacy support staff who has undergone limited training that allows them to order and dispense medicines, in addition to the role performed by a medicines counter assistant.
Dispensing doctor	A practitioner, typically in a rural area, who is licensed to dispense medicines to patients who live more than 1 mile from their nearest pharmacy.

Dispensing error	An error in the dispensing of a medication.
Dispersible	Describes a dosage form, usually a tablet, that breaks down into small particles in water and forms a suspension of those particles.
Dissolution	The kinetic process in which the molecules of a solid dissolve in a solvent such as the gastric fluid.
Domiciliary visit	Visit to a patient's home to provide a service, for example a medication review carried out in a patient's home would be a domiciliary medication review.
Dosage	The prescribed amount of medicine, including the dose (amount) and the timing (e.g. two tablets three times a day).
Dose	The amount of medication that a patient should take (e.g. one tablet).
Doubling-up	The process used when combining a small amount of one ingredient with a larger amount of another in order to ensure even distribution.
Drug chart	The prescription chart used in a hospital; this is a record of the medication that a patient is prescribed during their hospital stay. Each drug order is signed by a doctor (or other authorised prescriber) and a nurse signs the drug chart each time a medicine is administered. A pharmacist signs the drug chart and endorses it with additional instructions, an indication of where the medicine is available from (such as 'stock on the ward', 'patient's own', or the number of dose units supplied by the pharmacist) and the date.
Drug order	In a hospital setting, this refers to a prescription written for an individual patient on a drug chart.
Duration	The length of time for which a patient will take a medication (e.g. 1 week).
Duty of care	A legal obligation to provide a reasonable standard of care to a patient when providing a service such as dispensing a prescription or counter prescribing.
Efficacy	The ability to produce a desired outcome. In terms of medicines, this refers to the ability of a medicine to produce the desired therapeutic outcome.
Elective admission	Routine planned admission to hospital, usually for surgery or other planned treatment.
Elixir	A sweet-tasting liquid preparation of a pharmaceutical product. Similar to a linctus, but containing less alcohol.
Embrocation	A medicinal liquid that is rubbed into the skin to relieve muscular stiffness and pain.
Emergency admission	Non-routine unplanned admission to hospital for an illness or injury (e.g. by ambulance or through the Emergency department).
Emergency department	Point of contact for emergency care provided by hospitals (formerly called A&E – Accident and Emergency).
Emergency supply	A supply of a medication usually taken by a patient that is provided by a pharmacist in an emergency where the patient does not have a prescription.
Emollient	A substance composed of fat or oil that soothes and softens the skin.
Emulsion	A mixture of oil and water, generally of a milky or cloudy appearance.
Endoscope	An instrument that is inserted into the body to view internal parts.
Enema	Liquid or foam dosage form that is administered via the rectum.
Enhanced service	The highest tier of service provision under the new Pharmacy Contract, which contains services that can be commissioned from community

	pharmacies by primary care trusts according to the needs of the local population.
Enteral	Administration of food or medication via the gastrointestinal tract.
Enteric coating	A special coating applied to tablets or capsules to protect the dosage form from degradation by stomach acid or to protect the stomach from irritant drugs. The coating is susceptible to degradation by the alkaline environment of the small intestine, where the drug is released and absorbed.
Enterostomal tube	A tube that runs from an opening in the skin of the abdomen into the stomach or jejunum.
Enzyme enhancement	Increase in the ability of enzymes to carry out their required function.
Enzyme inhibition	Prevention or reduction of an enzyme's ability to carry out a process, as a result of the interaction of some substance with the enzyme.
Epidural	Administration of a medication (usually an anaesthetic) by injection into the epidural space around the spinal column via a lumbar puncture.
Essential service	The lowest tier of service provision under the new Pharmacy Contract, which contains services which must be provided by all community pharmacies.
Excipient	A biologically inactive substance used as a carrier for the active ingredients of a medication (i.e. the drug). Excipients are included in a formulation for their specific properties such as bulking, improving powder flow, solubility, disintegration and mechanical strength.
Expiry date	The date after which a drug product should not be used or taken. The period of time between manufacture and the expiry date depends on the stability of the product.
Extemporaneous preparation	The preparation of a medicinal product from individual ingredients within a pharmacy in response to a prescription for an individual patient. Products are either prepared to recipes from the standard formularies (e.g. *British Pharmacopeia*) or to recipes written by the prescriber. These are unlicensed products.
Food and Drug Administration (FDA)	The organisation that grants marketing authorisations in the USA.
Final check	The final check that a pharmacist (or appropriately qualified technician if a prescription has already been clinically checked by a pharmacist) makes to ensure that the dispensed medicinal product is the same as that requested by a prescriber on a prescription.
First-pass effect	Metabolism in the liver of a drug that has been absorbed via the gastrointestinal tract and is carried directly to the liver via the portal vein, before reaching the target organ. Efficacy may be reduced by first-pass effect (also known as first-pass metabolism); some drugs are activated by this process (e.g. tramadol).
Formulary	A list of medications that are approved for prescription/supply in a local area, for example within a hospital trust.
Formulation	The quantities and sources of ingredients used to make a product; the act, process, or result of formulating or reducing to a formula.
Foundation hospital trust	Management structure for highly performing hospitals that provides greater independence and financial control compared with NHS acute trusts.
Frequency	How often a patient should take their medication (e.g. twice a day).

Friability	The resistance of a product to being broken into smaller pieces by mechanical force such as a tablet breaking in a tablet jar.
General Medical Services contract	The contract under which general practitioners provide a medical service within the NHS.
General practice	The team of general practitioners and staff such as practice nurses, practice pharmacists, and receptionists who provide primary health care.
General practitioner	A doctor who practises in a primary care environment (the general practice).
General sales list (GSL)	A list of medicinal products that are available for sale without the supervision of a registered pharmacist; however, if they are being sold from a registered pharmacy, a pharmacist must be present.
Generic medication	Medication known by its official (non-brand) name. This name is not protected by trademark (e.g. propranolol slow-release (generic) vs Inderal (branded)).
GP fundholder	General practice that has responsibility for its own budget.
Granulation	Process by which a primary powder of drug and excipients adheres by the addition of a solvent(s) to form larger multiparticulates called granules. Granules usually have superior flow properties to powders.
Haematology	The clinical speciality or area of the hospital where patients with diseases of the blood are treated.
Haematoma	A collection of blood under the skin that forms a swelling.
Half-life	The time taken for the concentration of drug in the plasma to decrease by 50%.
Healthcare Commission	Independent watchdog that oversees the provision of health care and public health services by the NHS; accountable to the Secretary of State for Health.
Health screening	Testing members of the general public for the presence of common conditions such as diabetes, raised cholesterol or hypertension.
High-risk prescription	A prescription where there is a high risk of injury to a patient if the medication is administered as prescribed.
Hypertension	High blood pressure.
Independent prescriber	Non-medical prescriber who has undergone a structured training programme that allows them to prescribe medications within the constraints of their clinical knowledge and professional judgement (includes pharmacists and nurses amongst others).
Independent sector treatment centre (ISTC)	Privately run treatment centre commissioned by a primary care trust to provide services (such as minor surgery) that have traditionally been associated with long waiting times when provided by hospitals.
Infusion	A fluid injected slowly over a long period of time via the intravenous or intraperitoneal route (more than 5 minutes; may last for many hours). Infusions are usually large volumes of fluid.
Inpatient	A patient who stays in hospital for one or more nights.
Integrated care pathway	A flow diagram which allows the care provided to a patient to be recorded on a document that provides evidence-based practice guidelines for patient care.
Intentional non-adherence	Non-adherence in which a patient chooses not to take their medication according to the prescribed regimen.

Interaction	The effect of a medication on the body; the effect of a reaction (chemical or physical) between two or more medications (drug–drug interaction) or a medication and a food substance (food–drug interaction).
Intercellular matrix	The substance around cells of the body, composed of tissue fluid and structural macromolecules such as collagens and glycoproteins; also referred to as interstitial fluid.
International normalised ratio (INR)	A measure of how well a person's blood clots, used to determine how much anticoagulant (blood-thinning medication) a patient should take.
Intervention	*See* Prescription intervention.
Intra-articular	Administration of medication by injection into a joint.
Intradermal	Administration of medication by injection into the layer of the skin known as the dermis.
Intramuscular	Administration of a medication by injection into a muscle.
Intra-osseous (IO)	Administration of a medication by injection into a bone (only used in children under 6 years of age).
Intraperitoneal (IP)	Administration of a medication by injection or infusion into the abdominal cavity (the peritoneum).
Intrathecal (IT)	Administration of medication by injection into the cerebrospinal fluid surrounding the spinal column.
Intravenous (IV)	Administration of a medication by injection into a vein.
Isotonic	Describes a fluid that contains the same concentration of salts as the plasma.
Jejunum	A section of the gastrointestinal tract; the first part of the small intestine.
Leading question	A question that guides the response of the person answering, such as 'Is your inhaler brown?' *See* Closed question.
Licensed dose	The dose (or dose range) specified in the marketing authorisation.
Licensed indication	The clinical condition(s) specified in the marketing authorisation.
Linctus	A sweet-tasting liquid preparation of a pharmaceutical product; similar to an elixir, but less sweet and containing more alcohol.
Liniment	A medicinal preparation meant for external use that is thinner in consistency than an ointment (from the Latin *linere:* to anoint).
Local effect	The effect of a medication when it occurs in the area surrounding the point of administration, rather than having a systemic effect (i.e. spreading through the body via the circulation and affecting many areas).
Lotion	An oil-in-water emulsion; a powdered, insoluble solid held in suspension.
Lubricant	An oily or slippery substance that reduces friction.
Lumbar puncture	Insertion of a hollow needle into the spinal cord in the lower back.
Magnetic flea	A plastic-coated magnetic object that can be placed in a container of liquid and used with a magnetic stirring device to combine other materials into the liquid.
Marketing authorisation (MA)	The licence granted to a pharmaceutical manufacturer by the MHRA when they provide sufficient evidence to satisfy the regulatory agencies of the safety and efficacy of a medicinal product. Ideally, only products with an MA should be supplied to patients, unless there is no licensed alternative.
Medical gases	Gases used to produce a therapeutic effect, such as oxygen, nitrous oxide ('laughing gas', used as an anaesthetic and analgesic, especially during labour) and gaseous anaesthetics, such as sevoflurane.

Medical record	A record of a patient's care, including details of consultations with health professionals, current and past treatments, and current and past illnesses. At present, separate records are held in hospitals and general practices.
Medicated water	A water extraction of a solid medicinal substance.
Medication error	An error in the provision of a medication to the patient; can occur at any stage in the medication use process (prescribing, dispensing, administering or monitoring).
Medication history	A record of the medication which a patient takes at home, including prescribed medication, medication bought OTC, herbal and other complementary therapies, and vitamin supplements. In addition, this record should also include medication which has recently been stopped.
Medication review	The process of reviewing a patient's medication, either with or without the patient present, to assess whether the medication is safe and appropriate to continue.
Medicinal chemistry	The design, synthesis and development of pharmaceutical drugs. Medicinal chemistry lies between chemistry and pharmacology.
Medicinal product	A chemical with a medicinal use which has been formulated to enable it to be taken by humans or animals (as appropriate).
Medicinal substance	A chemical which has a medicinal use.
Medicines and Healthcare products Regulatory Agency (MHRA)	The organisation in the UK that deals with the licensing and regulation of medicines and medical devices; marketing authorisations for new drugs are granted by the MHRA.
Medicines counter assistant	Member of the pharmacy support staff who has undergone limited training that allows them to sell over-the-counter medicines within the constraints of a protocol.
Medicines information (MI)	The team within a hospital pharmacy who answer queries from health professionals and patients about medicines.
Medicines management	The systematic provision of medicines therapy through a partnership effort between patients and health professionals to deliver best patient outcome at minimum cost.
Medicines use review (MUR)	A review of how a patient takes their medicines at home, undertaken by a community pharmacist with the patient present.
Meniscus	The curved surface of the liquid at the fill point of a glass container; the fluid level next to the glass is higher than in the centre and the level in a container is read from the centre of the meniscus.
Mental health trusts	Provide specialist health and social care to patients with mental health problems.
Minor ailment/illness	An illness that does not have serious health implications for a patient and can be safely treated by a community pharmacist with the range of medications available over the counter.
Minor ailment scheme	A scheme that allows patients to obtain treatments for minor ailments (such as hay fever, or cold and flu symptoms) free of charge from a pharmacy without a prescription from their GP.
Mixture	A combination of two or more substances that have not combined chemically and that can be separated by physical means.
Monitoring	The process of assessing the response of a patient to a medicine or other treatment.
Morbidity	An illness or disease.

'Morning-after pill'	A one-off dose of progesterone given to women within 72 hours of unprotected sex to reduce the risk of an unwanted pregnancy (also known as emergency hormonal contraception).
Mortality	Death.
Mortar (and pestle)	A bowl-shaped vessel in which substances can be ground (and mixed with a pestle).
Multiple-item prescription	A prescription that has more than one prescription item on it.
Mydriatic	A medication that dilates the pupil.
Nanotechnology	Control of matter at the molecular level, in scales smaller than 1 micrometre, normally 1–100 nanometres, and the fabrication of devices within that size range.
Narrow therapeutic index	A narrow drug plasma concentration range at which a drug is effective. At concentrations below this range the drug may not be effective; it is likely to exert toxic effects at concentrations above the therapeutic range. Some drugs used to treat epilepsy (e.g. phenytoin) have a narrow therapeutic range.
Nasogastric (NG) tube	A tube from the nose into the stomach for administering liquids or medications.
Nasojejunal (NJ) tube	A tube from the nose into the jejunum (the first part of the small intestine, just below the stomach) for administering liquids or medications.
National Institute for Health and Clinical Excellence (NICE)	Special Health Authority that makes recommendations on which treatments should be used in the NHS on the basis of their cost-effectiveness.
National Service Framework (NSF)	National standard of care for the treatment of a specific patient group, such as the elderly, children, and patients with heart disease.
Near miss	An error that is identified before causing harm to a patient (or having the potential to cause harm to a patient).
Net ingredient cost (NIC)	The cost of each ingredient contained on a prescription.
New chemical entity	A drug molecule that is new and chemically unique (i.e. does not contain an active part that has previously been licensed by a government agency, such as the MHRA or FDA).
NHS acute trusts	Management structure for hospitals (or groups of hospitals) that are commissioned by primary care trusts to provide acute health care.
Non-adherence	Describes a situation in which patient does not take their medication (or follow other recommendations about their health) as they have previously agreed to during consultation with a health professional. This is a less negative term than non-compliance.
Non-clinical speciality	An area of pharmacy that does not involve direct patient contact on wards or in hospital clinics, such as management and sterile and non-sterile production.
Non-compliance	Describes a situation in which a patient does not take their medication (or follow other health advice) as directed by a health professional. This is a negative term implying disobedience on the part of the patient. The preferred term is non-adherence (described above).
Non-concordance	Describes a consultation where a patient and health professional cannot agree on decision about the patient's care.
Non-sterile production	The area within a hospital pharmacy where non-sterile medicinal products (such as creams and ointments) are made in a clean environment.
Nostrum	A favourite but untested remedy for problems or evils, traditionally formulated by a pharmacist.

Oncology	The clinical speciality relating to study and treatment of cancer.
Onset of action	The point at which a drug starts to exert its therapeutic effect. This is usually the time from when the dose was taken.
Open and fair approach	An approach which, when an error occurs, encourages staff to explore why the error occurred and to report this centrally, to help organisations learn from the experience. Instead of focusing on the individual directly responsible for the error, an open and fair approach focuses on the factors that contributed to the error, such as the working environment and staff resources.
Open question	A question that has no right or wrong response and therefore usually encourages the person answering to give a detailed answer (e.g. 'Tell me about. . .').
Optimising pack sizes	The process of ensuring that prescriptions are written for the number of dose units contained in an original pack of medication. This avoids pharmacists having to split original packs of medication.
Oral	Administration of a medication by swallowing.
Oral drops	A liquid formulation of a pharmaceutical product, usually at a high concentration, to reduce the volume needed to be taken by the patient.
Oral liquid	A liquid formulation of a pharmaceutical product.
Organisational structure	The management structure of an organisation which influences the working conditions of staff.
Orthopaedics	The clinical speciality that deals with fractured bones and bone diseases.
Osmotic effect	In the context of pharmacy, this is the effect of a medicine with a high concentration, such as lactulose, to draw water into the gastrointestinal tract, and therefore increase the volume of the gastrointestinal contents.
Osmotic potential	The capability of a solution to draw water into it when divided from another solution by a semi-permeable membrane, such as a cellular membrane, or the mucous membrane of the intestinal wall.
Outpatient	A patient who attends hospital during the day but does not stay overnight (e.g. for minor surgery or specialist clinics).
Over-the-counter (OTC) sale	The supply of a GSL or 'P' medicine that can be sold from a registered pharmacy under the supervision of a registered pharmacist (*see* separate entries for definitions of GSL and 'P' medicines).
Palette knife	A blunt knife with a flexible steel blade and no sharpened cutting edge, used for combining ingredients of creams or ointments on a ceramic slab.
Parenteral nutrition	The administration of nutrients intravenously.
Patent (drug)	A licence that restricts the manufacture of a particular drug product to the company that registers the patent for a set period of time (e.g. 10 years).
Patented remedy	A medicine containing one or more ingredients, designed by a particular pharmacist and protected by law from reproduction by other parties.
Paternalistic	Treating patients in a 'fatherly manner', particularly making decisions for patients without giving them the opportunity to contribute to the decision or to take any responsibility for the decision.
Patient Advisory and Liaison Service (PALS)	Provides a point of contact for patients to comment on the care they have received within the NHS. Also provides information about NHS services and support to patients and their carers. Acute NHS trusts and primary care trusts will have a PALS.

Patient counselling	The process of advising patients about their medicines, including what the medicine is for, how and when to take it, what side-effects to expect and what to do if they occur.
Patient group direction (PGD)	A written instruction that allows the legal sale, supply or administration of a medicine to a patient (or group of patients) in a clearly defined clinical situation without the necessity for a legal prescription.
Patient information leaflet (PIL)	An information sheet supplied with a medication which informs patients about what the medication is for, how it should be taken, and what side-effects might occur.
Patient medication record (PMR)	An electronic record of the medication that has been dispensed for an individual patient by a pharmacy.
Patient pack	Usually a 28-day supply of a medication in a blister pack, also containing a patient information leaflet (defined above).
Payment by results (PBR)	The process by which healthcare providers are paid for the services they provide (e.g. surgical operations; each service is assigned a tariff (the average cost of the service)).
Peak flow	A measure of how fast a patient can blow air out of their lungs.
Percutaneous	Through the skin.
Percutaneous endoscopic gastrostomy (PEG)	Insertion of a feeding tube from an opening in the skin of the abdomen into the stomach; the abbreviation PEG is also used to refer to the tube itself.
Percutaneous endoscopic jejunostomy (PEJ)	Insertion of a feeding tube that goes from an opening in the skin of the abdomen into the jejunum; the abbreviation PEJ is also used to refer to the tube itself.
Perfumes	Scents added to pharmaceutical products to mask unpleasant odours.
Peritonitis	Inflammation of the peritoneal wall (the wall surrounding the abdominal cavity), often caused by an infection.
Pestle (mortar and pestle)	A club-shaped hand tool for grinding and mixing substances (in a mortar).
Pharmaceutical care	The responsible provision of drug therapy for the purpose of achieving definite outcomes that improve a patient's quality of life.
Pharmaceutics	The science of dosage form design (i.e. the processes of turning a new chemical entity into an efficacious medicine that can be administered safely).
Pharmacokinetics	The study of the fate of substances such as drugs within the body. The main phases are absorption, distribution, metabolism and excretion (sometimes abbreviated to ADME).
Pharmacology	The science of the properties of drugs and their effects on the body.
Pharmacopoeia	A pharmacopeia (literally, the art of the drug compounder) is, in its modern technical sense, a book containing directions for the identification of samples and the preparation of compounded medicines, published by the authority of a government or medical or pharmaceutical society.
Pharmacy Contract	The contract under which community pharmacies provide a pharmaceutical service to patients under the NHS. This contract includes three tiers of service provision: essential, advanced and enhanced.
Pharmacy support staff	Members of the pharmacy team who have undergone varied levels of training to allow them to perform tasks traditionally undertaken by pharmacists.

Pharmacy technician	Member of the pharmacy support staff who has completed more extensive training than other pharmacy support staff, allowing them to perform a wide range of tasks traditionally undertaken by pharmacists; pharmacy technicians are encouraged to register with the Royal Pharmaceutical Society of Great Britain.
Phase	A distinct state of matter in a system (e.g. the solid phase, the liquid phase).
Physicochemical characteristics	The particular profile of physical and chemical behaviour associated with a compound (e.g. melting point, solubility, ionisation characteristics).
Pills	A medicinal or other active substance mixed with binder powders and pressed into a (spherical) tablet form.
Placebo	A substance that has no known biological activity, but may help relieve a condition because the patient has faith in its ability to do so (the so-called placebo effect). Wherever possible, new drugs are compared with a placebo in clinical trials; the placebo tablet will appear identical to the tablets containing the active drug.
Plasma concentration	The level of a substance in the blood plasma.
Plaster	A paste-like mixture applied to a part of the body for healing or cosmetic purposes.
Polymorph	A solid, such as a drug, that shares its chemical composition with another material but is composed of a different crystal lattice or form. The polymorph solid will have different properties such as solubility and lattice energies.
Polypharmaceuticals/ polypharmacy	The use of more than one clinically justified medication concurrently.
'POM to P' switch	Deregulation of a medicinal product that has previously been licensed for prescription only use to a pharmacy medicine, available for sale over the counter.
Powder	A medicinal substance consisting of ground, pulverised or otherwise finely dispersed solid particles.
Practice-based commissioning (PBC)	The process by which general practices purchase healthcare services for the general population that they serve.
Pre-registration placement	A 12-month period of vocational training undertaken as part of the training to become a pharmacist. The type of training is outlined in criteria from the Royal Pharmaceutical Society of Great Britain. Pharmacy students undertake the training either in a 1 year block after graduation (4 years at university and 1 year's training 'on the job') or as two 6 month blocks integrated into the undergraduate education (5 years in total).
Prescribing	The process of choosing and writing a prescription for a medicine to give to a patient.
Prescribing errors	An error in the prescription of a medication.
Prescription chart	*See* Drug chart.
Prescription intervention	The process by which a pharmacist requests that a prescriber change a prescription in order to make the prescription legal, to reduce the cost of the prescription, or to ensure that the prescribed medication is safe and effective for a patient to take.
Prescription item	A single named medicinal product (or appliance) on a prescription.

Prescription laboratory	A room or area of the dispensary dedicated to making up special products on the order of a physician.
Prescription-only Medicine (POM)	A medicinal product that can only be supplied in response to a prescription written by an authorised prescriber.
Preventable drug-related morbidity (PDRM)	An adverse event caused by an error in the provision of a medication to a patient where the patient harm was foreseeable and avoidable.
Primary care	The first point of contact with health care for the general public (e.g. general practice surgeries, dentists, nurses, opticians, pharmacists).
Primary care trust (PCT)	One of 152 geographic areas that provide local management of health care and commission health services. PCTs are accountable to the strategic health authorities.
Primary non-adherence	Non-adherence (defined above) in which a patient does not have a prescription dispensed.
Primary packaging	Packaging material that comes into direct contact with a medicinal product.
Private prescription	A prescription that is not written on an official NHS prescription form and is therefore not paid for by the NHS.
Private prescription register	A record of private prescriptions (and the individual items on these) dispensed by a pharmacy.
Privy Council	A body that advises the head of state. In the UK, the Privy Council is composed of all the members of the Cabinet, former cabinet ministers, and other distinguished persons appointed by the sovereign. Its functions include granting royal charters and acting as a court of appeal from British courts in oversees territories.
Probing question	A question that is intended to get more detailed information about something, such as 'How many times a day do you use your inhaler?' *See* Open question.
Product licence	The old name for a marketing authorisation.
Professional check	The check which a pharmacist makes to ensure that a prescription is legal and clinically appropriate for an individual patient, and that the dispensed medicinal product is the same as that requested by the prescriber.
Professional fee	A payment made to a pharmacy for dispensing a prescription item on an NHS prescription.
Prophylaxis	The use of a medicinal product or other form of treatment with the intention of avoiding a future illness, for example taking medication to combat malaria before, during and after travel to countries known to have a malaria problem.
Proprietary remedy	A remedy to which the manufacturer has exclusive rights, usually marketed under a name that is registered as a trademark.
Public health	The health needs of the population as a whole (as opposed to individuals). Public health usually refers to the delivery of services targeted at preventing disease, such as smoking cessation.
Qualitative testing	Testing the quality of a substance or product, for instance the purity of a medicine.
Quality and Outcomes Framework (QOF)	Part of the contract that employs general practitioners within the NHS, providing financial incentives to general practices for the provision of excellent patient care.
Quality assurance	The provision of evidence that an item or product conforms with the established technical requirements.

Quality control	The inspection, analysis and action required to ensure the quality of a product.
Quantitative testing	Testing the amount, or quantity, of a substance in a product.
Rectal administration (PR (*per rectum*))	Administration of a medication via the rectum (back passage).
Register of Pharmaceutical Chemists	This document, held and controlled by the Royal Pharmaceutical Society of Great Britain, is a statutory database that is updated on an ongoing basis throughout the year, with the prime purpose of providing assurance to the public that pharmacists in practice are registered health professionals who fulfil the requirements of health, character and education, and are bound by the profession's code of ethics.
Renal failure	A medical condition in which the kidney(s) is no longer able to work at an optimal level. This can be acute (where it occurs suddenly) or chronic (where it is a longstanding condition).
Repeat dispensing	The process by which patients can collect medicines that are prescribed for long-term use, direct from the pharmacy, without the need to collect a prescription from their GP each time (as is the case with repeat prescribing).
Repeat prescription	A prescription for a medication that a patient is taking over a long period of time, which they can request from their general practice surgery without needing to see the doctor. Repeat prescriptions are authorised for a limited time period or number of issues, after which a patient should be reviewed by their general practitioner (or other prescriber) to ensure that it is appropriate to continue taking the medication.
Reservoir of drug	An area in the body where a drug accumulates before being dispersed throughout the body. This may happen in the skin, when the drug being delivered by a patch passes into the skin more quickly than it is dispersed by the blood supply.
Retailing	The process of selling goods to customers.
Reye's syndrome	A rare condition that predominantly occurs in young children following a viral infection. Patients initially have severe persistent vomiting and fever, followed by outbursts of wild behaviour, which progresses into convulsions and finally death. It is known to be associated with aspirin, particularly in children.
Risk factors	Factors (such as another disease or illness or behaviour such as smoking) that increase the risk of a patient developing a medical condition.
Risk management	The process of assessing whether something can go wrong, how likely it will go wrong, how severe the consequences might be, and how the unwanted outcome can be avoided.
Risk–benefit analysis	The process of assessing the risks and benefits of an action or treatment and deciding what to do in light of the balance between the two.
Royal Charter of Incorporation	A Charter is an authority directly from the monarch for a body to take certain powers. A Charter of Incorporation enables a body to function as a corporation (i.e. a large company or group of companies authorised to act as a single entity and recognised as such in law). The Royal Pharmaceutical Society of Great Britain operates under a Charter of Incorporation.

Royal Pharmaceutical Council	The Royal Pharmaceutical Council governs the Royal Pharmaceutical Society of Great Britain and is responsible for deciding on policy and practice relating to the society.
Royal Pharmaceutical Society of Great Britain (RPSGB)	The professional and governing body for pharmacists and pharmacy technicians in Great Britain.
Secondary (acute) care	Care provided by hospitals.
Secondary non-adherence	Non-adherence (defined above) in which a patient has a prescription dispensed but does not take the medication according to the directions agreed with the health professional.
Secondary packaging	Packaging material that encloses the primary packaging and does not come into direct contact with the medicinal product.
Secretary of State for Health	Senior government minister in charge of the Department of Health.
Sedate	Put a patient to sleep, or otherwise calm them, using a medication such as a benzodiazepine.
Selected list	A list of medications that can be prescribed on an NHS prescription for patients with a restricted list of conditions.
'Sick day rules'	Guidance given to diabetic patients on how to adjust their insulin dose to help maintain control of their blood glucose when they are ill.
Sick role	The role that a patient takes when they are unwell. The sick role means that they no longer have to perform their usual tasks, but in return they must make every effort to get well again (e.g. by taking medication).
Side-effects	Unanticipated effects of a medication – can be beneficial or harmful.
Signed order	A request to purchase a prescription-only medicine or a Schedule 1 poison.
Signposting	Referring patients to the most appropriate health or social care provider in order to reduce the inappropriate use of health and social care services.
Single electronic patient record	A single electronic record of a patient's medical and medication history available online. Health professionals will be able to access the information that they need in order to deliver effective care to patients from this record (not yet in existence at the time of writing).
Solubility	A chemical property referring to the ability for a given substance (the solute) to dissolve in a solvent.
Special health authority	An organisation that provides a range of centralised services to the NHS in England, for example (NICE, defined above).
Standard operating procedure (SOP)	A protocol that describes how (and by whom) a task, such as dispensing a medicinal product, should be carried out.
Sterile production	The area within a hospital pharmacy where sterile medicinal products (such as injections and eye drops) are made in a very clean environment to avoid contamination with bacteria or other microbes.
Sterility	The absence of pathogenic organisms.
Stock list	List of stock that is kept within the pharmacy.
Stoma	A surgically created opening from an area inside the body to the outside. For example, a colostomy is an opening from the colon through the abdominal wall to the outside the body.
Strategic health authority (SHA)	One of ten geographic areas that provide local management and strategic direction for the NHS, accountable to the Department of Health.

Strength	The amount of drug contained in a given dosage unit (e.g. a 50 mg tablet, or a 5 mg/mL liquid).
Subarachnoid space	The space between two of the three membranes covering the brain and spinal cord, which is filled with cerebrospinal fluid.
Subcutaneous (SC) injection	An injection from a needle placed underneath the skin (i.e. into the subcutaneous connective tissue).
Sublingual (SL)	Administration of a medication by placing it underneath the tongue.
Substance misuse	The administration of a substance by a person for purposes other than a therapeutic effect (e.g. solvent abuse, excessive alcohol intake, heroin addiction).
Sub-therapeutic dose	A dose of medication that is too low to produce the desired therapeutic effect.
Supplementary prescriber	A non-medical prescriber who has undergone a structured training programme that allows them to prescribe medications within the constraints of a clinical management plan agreed by the patient, their doctor and the supplementary prescriber (includes pharmacists and nurses amongst other others).
Suppository	A solid dosage form that is administered via the rectal route.
Suspension	A solid dosage form suspended in a liquid, usually water.
Symptomatic relief	Relief of symptoms of an illness or disease rather than treating the underlying condition.
Synovial fluid	Fluid within a joint that provides lubrication and nutrition of the joint.
Systemic circulation	The circulation that supplies blood to all parts of the body except the lungs.
Systemic effect	A generalised effect of a drug throughout the body, compared with a local effect which is restricted to the area of the body where the drug is delivered.
Syrup	A liquid dosage form containing a high percentage of sugar.
Targeted delivery	Where a drug molecule is modified (such as by association with a polymer) to preferentially target a specific site of action (e.g. a tumour).
The Society	A commonly used term that refers to the Royal Pharmaceutical Society of Great Britain.
Therapeutic concentration	The concentration of a drug in the blood plasma required for therapeutic effect.
Therapeutic decision	Making a decision about how to treat a patient, based on evidence, experience and the therapies available.
Therapeutic failure	A therapeutic failure occurs when treatment does not have the desired effect. In the case of medication, this might be because the prescribed dose is too low, the patient is not taking the medication or is taking it incorrectly, or an interaction occurs.
Therapeutic index	The ratio between the toxic dose and the therapeutic dose of a drug, used as a measure of the relative safety of the drug for a particular treatment.
Therapeutic response	When a positive clinical change is seen after the administration of a medicine (e.g. an antibiotic causing a reduction in bacterial load).
Therapeutic objective	The result desired when a drug is taken by a patient.
Therapeutics	The branch of medicine concerned with the treatment of disease with medicinal products (as opposed to surgery).
Tincture	A solution prepared by steeping or soaking plant materials in alcohol and water.

Topical	Administration of a medication by placing it on the skin or a mucous membrane.
Toxicology	The study of adverse effects (toxicity) of chemicals on living organisms.
Treatment regimen	The medication(s) (or other forms of therapy) that are recommended or prescribed to treat a patient's condition.
Trituration	The grinding of powders in a mortar with a pestle, before combining to make a cream, ointment or other pharmaceutical product.
Unguent	A soothing preparation spread on sores, burns, irritations or other topical injuries; an ointment. It is usually delivered as a semi-solid paste and is often oily to suspend the medication or other active ingredients.
Unintentional non-adherence	Non-adherence (defined above) in which a patient either forgets, or is unable, to take their medication according to the prescribed regimen.
Unlicensed dose	A dose of a licensed medication that is outside the dose range specified in the marketing authorisation.
Unlicensed indication	A clinical use of a medicinal product that is not included in the marketing authorisation.
Unlicensed medicine	A medicinal product that has not been granted a marketing authorisation.
Veterinary medicinal product	A medication used to treat animals.
Viscosity	A measure of the ease with which a liquid can be poured or stirred. The higher the viscosity, the less easily a liquid pours.
Ward round	When doctors and/or other health professionals review the patients on a ward.
Yellow Card Scheme	The system used by patients and health professionals to report suspected adverse drug reactions to the Medicines and Healthcare products Regulatory Agency (MHRA).

Index